Hormones, Health, and Happiness

A Natural Medical Formula for Rediscovering Youth

By Steven F. Hotze, M.D.

with Kelly Griffin

Published by Advantage Media Group
Charleston, SC

Distributed by Advantage Media Group

For ordering information or special discounts for bulk purchases, please contact Advantage Media Group, advantagefamily.com, 843-414-5600

Library of Congress Control Number: 2013930396

ISBN 978-159932-399-2

Part of the Tree Neutral® program, which offsets the number of trees consumed in the production and printing of this book by taking proactive steps, such as planting trees in direct proportion to the number of trees used: www.treeneutral.com

Printed in the United States of America on acid-free paper

10 11 12 13 14   10 9 8 7 6 5

Second Edition

TreeNeutral

ACKNOWLEDGMENTS

The success of any endeavor is directly dependent upon the collaborative work of many individuals. Every person has been shaped and molded by the influences of countless individuals during her or his lifetime. The influences of these individuals have contributed to who we are, to what we think and believe, and to what we accomplish.

So let me begin by crediting my mother, Margaret Hotze, for teaching me to abandon herd mentality, because, as she so often told me, "The herd is usually going in the wrong direction." Mom taught me to run away from the crowd, to do the right thing, and to be a leader. Unfortunately, I have not always heeded her advice, but when I have it has proven itself true. Her degree in journalism from the University of Texas has been used in serving as the editor of the *Life Advocate* newspaper for the past thirty years. Mom taught me to write. She has edited countless writings of mine over the years, starting with my term papers in high school. She is a voracious reader who founded Veritas, a Catholic bookstore in Houston, Texas. Mom has forgotten more than I will ever know.

My father, Ernest Hotze, was a most remarkable man, a great salesman, entrepreneur, and businessman who built a manufacturing business, Compressor Engineering Corporation (CECO), which currently employs over 150 individuals and is now run by four of my brothers. Dad worked his way through

Oklahoma University during the Depression working nights on an oil derrick. He was just as at ease with the presidents of major corporations as he was with the machinists or janitors working for him. Dad loved people. I remember him telling me that even the homeless person on the street was the apple of some mother's eye at one time. "Try to find something good in each person and focus on that," he often said. Dad was a success because he wanted everyone he knew to become successful and did whatever he could to help others achieve their goals.

Without the influence of my mother and father, I never would have been in a position to write this book. To both of them I will be forever grateful.

As a physician, when your family trusts you to provide them and their children with medical care, it is an honor. My six brothers and one sister have been my good friends and supporters throughout my life.

My wife, Janie, was a cheerleader for St. Thomas Catholic High School, which I attended in Houston, Texas. I fell in love with her during my senior year. We eloped before I entered college in 1968 and now have eight wonderful children and six grandchildren, with two more on the way. She has been the most devoted wife a man could ever dream of having. Janie threw herself into her role as mother, and she worked hard at it 24/7. She raised a great bunch of children who love her dearly. What a great testimony they are to her dedication and diligence! Janie has been my faithful supporter through thick and thin. There have been many lean times but she always remained hopeful, like a true cheerleader, even when it looked like the game was lost. She never lost faith in me, and because of that, she gave me the confidence to pull off many fourth-quarter comebacks in the "nick of time." Janie is loved and revered by all who know her, especially by our staff. Janie came off the sidelines during a crunch time for our practice in 1995 and served for seven years as our controller while raising a family. Had she not suited up at that time, the game probably would have been lost. I am so very proud of her for all of her accomplishments, the most important of which is our family. For Janie's contributions to improving the quality and enjoyment of my life I am so very thankful.

My children, Mary Beth, Catherine, Sarah, Paul, David, Patrick, Deborah, and Rebekah, have each contributed to my appreciation for the value of strong, supportive family relationships. I am grateful to them for the myriad of new experiences that they have brought into my life. In particular, I appreciate my son Paul, who has worked beside me in my enterprises, serving as vice president of marketing. His creative genius provided the impetus to reach tens of thousands of individuals who were looking for safe, effective, and natural solutions for their health problems. I am proud of his work and thankful that he was willing to join me in my endeavors.

Next to my father, the most influential man in my life was Charlie Casebolt. He led the Navigator Christian Ministry at the University of Texas, which helped college students develop their Christian lives. Charlie instilled in me the importance of building teamwork among like-minded individuals. The principles I learned from him continue to serve me today. Thank you, Charlie.

In September of 1990, a most remarkable woman, Monica Luedecke, walked into my office, seeking employment. She was the fourth person I hired after moving my office and transitioning into more natural approaches to health care. After interviewing her and offering her a position, I told Monica that if she would make herself indispensable she would always have a job with me. Over the past fourteen years she has done just that. She has gone from serving as chief cook and bottle washer in the front office to becoming executive vice president and chief of staff of three burgeoning enterprises: Hotze

Health & Wellness Center; Physicians Preference, our vitamin company; and Premier Pharmacy. She leads a combined staff of over ninety people. Monica took the personal initiative to develop the vitamin business and pharmacy from scratch while I was practicing medicine. She has been my mastermind ally, and without her organizational ability, our businesses would be mere shadows of what they are today. Monica is an outstanding businesswoman whose advice and counsel have been invaluable to me and everyone whom she serves in her leadership position. Monica has played an integral role in helping me write and edit this book. Without her persistence it would never have been accomplished. I will forever remain grateful to her for her friendship and support.

Our leadership team encouraged me to write this book years ago. It is a privilege to work with such an outstanding group of individuals who are committed to serving one another and to serving our guests as we lead the Wellness Revolution and build the finest health and wellness businesses in the world.

It has been my privilege and honor to be associated with the finest staff members in the world. These women and men are dedicated and passionate about providing extraordinary hospitality and medical care. Their positive, enthusiastic, and caring personalities provide an environment that cultivates hope and instills a sense of well-being in each of our guests.

My colleagues Dr. David Sheridan and Dr. Donald Ellsworth have carried the load of evaluating and treating our guests during the past two years so that I could focus my attention on completing this book. Both of these gentlemen have been willing to challenge conventional medical thinking and adopt a more natural approach to health and wellness. I admire and appreciate them.

Dr. Jack Healey encouraged me to enter medical school and championed my application. He was instrumental in my acceptance to the University of Texas Medical School at Houston in 1972. Without his help I might now be a homebuilder, which was my second choice of professions.

During my internship at St. Joseph's Hospital in Houston, Texas, I came under the tutelage of Dr. Herb Fred, the ultimate clinician. Dr. Fred always asked his students, "Why? Why? Why?" He taught me to question everything, to search for the answers, and to ably defend my positions. He was an unconventional thinker, just as every successful person is.

In 1989, I joined the Pan American Allergy Society (PAAS), which is made up of an eclectic group of physicians who have chosen to take the road less traveled in order to help their patients restore their health. The members of this organization influenced me to travel with them through their lectures, teachings, and examples. These physicians have provided me with the practical knowledge to help thousands of my patients. To each of them I owe a debt of gratitude. Of all of them, Richard Mabray, M.D., an ob-gyn who discovered the relationship between allergies and thyroid disorders, has had the biggest impact in my medical practice. Ann Brey, the executive director of PAAS, has been the glue that has held this organization together for the past fifteen years. She registered me at the last minute for my first allergy conference in 1989 and encouraged me to teach and take leadership positions in this organization. I will always be grateful for the interest she has taken in me.

Kelly Griffin has faithfully served as my editor for this book. She has read, edited, reread, and reedited this book over the past year. Her recommendations have significantly improved its content. Her patience and dedication to this project have been just what the doctor ordered. Because of her extraordinary work, I am pleased to place her name on the front cover with mine.

Finally, I must commend my patients, who have been willing to make an investment in their health and wellness.

Their willingness to entrust me with their medical care humbles me. The discipline that they have exhibited in following my treatment regimen amazes me. The improvements that they have made in their health and wellness encourage me. It has been my honor and privilege to serve them and lead them onto the path of health and wellness.

The old adage "If momma ain't happy, ain't nobody happy" is really true. When a woman is suffering from a hormonal imbalance, it affects much more than her reproductive organs. It affects her mood, her energy, and her outlook on life, as well as her relationships with family members, friends, and coworkers. Louise, whose story will be told in this book, had no idea of the toll that her hormonal imbalance had taken in her life and in her relationships with loved ones until the proper balance was restored.

Not surprisingly, when I saw Louise for her follow-up visit after she had begun taking biologically identical hormones, her elation over finally feeling well was mixed with sadness and regret. "I reflected on my life over the past twenty years," she told me, "and then wrote my son a letter apologizing for being such an irritable, moody, depressed mother. He was five years old when I had my hysterectomy. I just wish I had known about natural progesterone then."

Faith has chosen me as an advocate of the truths which are laid down in this work . . .

I have abandoned the hope that the importance and the truth of the facts would make all conflict unnecessary.

—Ignaz Semmelweis, Hungarian physician (1818–1865)

Contents

CHAPTER 1
Creating Hormonal Harmony

Are you sick and tired of being sick and tired?

Are you weary of doctors who won't listen to you, don't understand you, and offer only prescription drugs as the solution to your health problems?

Are you frustrated with being told that your blood tests are "normal" and there is nothing wrong with you?

I understand how you feel. Daily at my clinic, I see women who have sought the care of numerous physicians for fatigue, weight gain, mood swings, menstrual irregularities, headaches, joint and muscle pain, loss of libido, and numerous other problems. They have had their blood drawn and their hormone levels measured, only to be told that no physical cause of their symptoms could be found.

A woman who is repeatedly told by her doctor that everything is "normal" even though she does not feel well is unlikely to get the personal attention and compassionate treatment that she deserves. Instead, she will be categorized as a hypochondriac, prescribed an antidepressant, or referred to a psychiatrist.

Initially, she may reject the idea of using antidepressants because she is still convinced that something within her body is not functioning correctly. But eventually, as her condition persists, she will comply with her doctor's wishes and take the drugs. When these drugs provide no relief, she may begin to consider that the doctor is right and that her problems are "all in her head." Even worse, she may conclude, as some women have revealed to me, that God is punishing her for her past sins.

If this is the way you feel, then please take note. Your health problems are not "all in your head." Your symptoms are very real and have a physical cause. You are not being punished by God. However, you may be suffering needlessly at the hands of unsympathetic physicians who do not have the time, the interest, or the training to determine the root cause of your problems.

The problems experienced by women during midlife are commonly a result of an imbalance in the female hormones and an overall decline in hormone production. The negative effects of this hormonal imbalance are not limited to the reproductive system. The female hormones play important roles throughout the body, in the heart, brain, muscles, bones, and other major organs and tissues.

The female hormones also interact with hormones produced by other glands, and an imbalance in levels of estrogen and progesterone adversely affects the production and use of these hormones. Fatigue, weight gain, mood and memory problems, insomnia, headaches, and menstrual disorders can all be traced back to various hormonal imbalances and deficiencies. One common result of female hormonal imbalance is hypothyroidism, or low thyroid function, which weakens the immune system and can trigger allergies, chemical sensitivities, and recurrent infections during midlife. Adrenal insufficiency often accompanies low thyroid function, worsening the problems of low energy, impaired immunity, and allergies.

Blood testing, which is a standard diagnostic tool of conventional medicine, is not the best way to diagnose hormonal problems or to assess whether the treatment of these problems is working. The most reliable indication of a hormonal problem is how a patient feels physically, mentally, and emotionally. Likewise, the most important criteria for evaluating the benefits of treatment are the resolution of symptoms and the overall improvement in a patient's well-being.

This approach, which entails listening to the patient's description of her problems and making a diagnosis based on this description, is a lost art in current medical practice. Today's physicians rely almost exclusively on laboratory tests in making diagnoses. While this may be necessary for certain diseases, it is not an effective or appropriate way to evaluate and treat the problems caused by hormonal imbalances and deficiencies that occur in midlife to both women and men.

FROM TREATING ILLNESS TO PROMOTING WELLNESS

Between 1976 and 1988, I practiced medicine conventionally, the way most physicians in this country do: I prescribed drugs. When a patient came into my office with allergies, I prescribed an antihistamine. For a patient who had high blood pressure, I prescribed an antihypertensive drug. If a patient suffered from anxiety, I prescribed an antianxiety medication. There was no end to the number of "antidotes" that could be prescribed to address one or another of my patients' symptoms. When the drugs I prescribed had bothersome side effects, other drugs could be prescribed to take care of those symptoms.

For an acute illness, such as strep throat or a sinus infection, the drug approach may be appropriate. However, few patients with chronic ailments ever really get well by taking drugs. How can they? Chronic illness and disease are not caused by deficiencies of prescription drugs. The causes are complex, relating to poor nutrition, lack of exercise, a stressful lifestyle, a weakened immune system, and declines in levels of hormones, to name only a few of the key contributing factors.

By the time I reached my thirteenth year as a practicing physician, I had lost my enthusiasm for my chosen profession. It was obvious that the drugs I had been prescribing for my patients' health problems were not making them feel better. In fact, in many cases, the drugs were making them feel worse. However, prescribing drugs is what I had been trained to do.

I simply didn't know another way to help my patients.

At this crucial juncture, when I was seriously contemplating walking away from medicine altogether, I had a seemingly chance encounter with an allergist. After hearing him talk with passion about the profession I no longer found gratifying, and listening to his successful case stories, I was inspired to seek training and education in the diagnosis and treatment of allergies. Although I didn't know it at the time, this was the beginning of a new phase of my career. From that point onward, medicine became an immensely enjoyable vocation for me. Finally, I was able to get to the root causes of many of my patients' illnesses and enable them to obtain and maintain optimal health.

The book you hold in your hands is actually two books in one. First, it is the story of my journey down the road less traveled, from mainstream physician to wellness practitioner. Second, and most important, it is a guidebook designed to help you begin your own journey down the road to optimal health and wellness.

In this book, you will learn about an eight-point treatment program developed to address the underlying causes of the most common health problems that occur in midlife. The components of this comprehensive program are:

1. Treatment of airborne allergies
2. Treatment of food allergies
3. Treatment of yeast overgrowth (candida)
4. Treatment of low thyroid function (hypothyroidism)

5. Natural hormone replacement in women and men
6. Treatment of adrenal fatigue
7. Nutritionally balanced eating program
8. Vitamin and mineral supplementation

All eight of the elements listed above are important to the optimal functioning of your cells, tissues, and organs and to how you feel physically, mentally, and emotionally. For example, consuming the right kinds and amounts of protein, carbohydrates, and fats can keep your energy levels steady throughout the day while helping you avoid the serious diseases that result from a lifetime of unhealthy food choices.

Nutritional supplements are much more than an insurance policy against deficiency diseases like scurvy and rickets. Studies have shown that taking optimal amounts of key nutrients, amounts that in some cases are much higher than the recommended daily allowance (RDA), can actually reduce your risk of cancer, heart disease, and a host of other illnesses and maladies.

Treating food and airborne allergies and eradicating yeast from the body can help rejuvenate the immune system, restore energy, and alleviate seemingly unrelated conditions like headaches, sinus and respiratory infections, asthma, digestive problems, and skin disorders.

However, of all of the elements outlined above, I have come to believe that the three that involve replenishing and balancing levels of key hormones are the most important to obtaining and maintaining optimal health and well-being.

Why are hormones so important? Quite simply, the aging process is the result of declining hormone levels. Levels of most hormones peak in our twenties and begin a slow, inexorable decline thereafter. As levels drop below their youthful peaks, you may begin to lose energy and gain weight. You may experience mood problems or have difficulty with thinking, concentration, and short-term memory. Your immune system is likely to become less efficient, leaving you vulnerable to infectious diseases. Restoring hormones to their optimal levels using natural, biologically identical hormones, is a safe, effective way to preserve vitality as you mature.

The key term in that sentence is "biologically identical." I am no fan of the counterfeit hormones manufactured by drug companies. These drugs are not identical to the hormones that are present naturally in the human body. In fact, in order to be patented, these drugs cannot be identical to your body's own hormones or to any other molecule that exists in nature. They must be chemically unique. This enables drug companies to have proprietary use of these drugs without competition and subsequently to reap huge profits from their sale. Women who take these artificial hormones pay the price, not just with their pocketbooks, but also with their health and well-being.

Because counterfeit hormones are not identical to the hormones produced by your body, they do not fit perfectly into the receptor sites in your body's cells. That is why these drugs can never restore optimal health. In fact, a wealth of research conducted over the past several decades clearly shows that, far from being age-defying wonder drugs, counterfeit female hormones such as Premarin, Provera, and Prempro may cause serious disease. Major studies, such as the Women's Health Initiative in the United States and the Million Women Study in Great Britain, have documented that these drugs increase the risk of life-threatening ailments such as breast cancer, heart attack, stroke, pulmonary embolism, and Alzheimer's disease.

Women today who are experiencing symptoms of hormonal imbalance or deficiency are given few options by conventional physicians. Some physicians continue to prescribe counterfeit hormones, despite their known dangers, insisting that the benefits outweigh the risks. Others have begun to prescribe antidepressants as the alternative to counterfeit hormones, as if mind-altering drugs are the solution to declining hormone levels. Still others have given up on the treatment of female hormone problems altogether and tell patients that they simply must learn to live with their symptoms.

However, there is a remarkably simple and safe alternative, which has received relatively little attention in the mainstream press. The alternative is the use of bioidentical hormones, formulated from plants and made identical to the estrogens, progesterone, and testosterone produced in the human body. Unlike counterfeit hormones, bioidentical hormones fit perfectly into the hormone receptors found in the cells of the body and produce natural, biological results without undesirable side effects.

Unfortunately, the major drug companies have no interest in biologically identical hormones because these hormones cannot be patented. Because drug companies are not interested in producing and marketing bioidentical hormones, most doctors have not been trained in their use and are unaware of the benefits of this type of therapy. After all, most physicians receive their continuing medical education at seminars and conferences sponsored by drug companies.

My staff and I have seen thousands of our patients get their lives back by following the comprehensive program outlined in this book. Because we have witnessed firsthand the dramatic improvement in health and wellness that can be obtained with the proper use of natural, bioidentical hormones, along with a healthy diet, nutritional supplementation, and the treatment of allergies and yeast, we believe it is our moral imperative to widely disseminate the information about our program.

I have written this book to give you information that you will not receive from the mainstream media, the medical establishment, or conventional physicians who are steeped in the "disease and drugs" model of medicine. My hope is that, once you have a better understanding of the root causes of your health problems, you will be inspired to find a doctor who can guide you onto the path to wellness. Most important, my deepest desire is to help you obtain and maintain health and wellness naturally so that you enjoy a better quality of life.

CHAPTER 2

Doctor, Am I a Hypochondriac?

When thirty-two-year-old Maggie came to see me, she was experiencing a host of medical problems that had arisen after the birth of her first child two years prior. Her menstrual cycles had become irregular, with her periods occurring as frequently as one to three weeks apart, lasting as long as seventeen days, and being accompanied by severe cramps. She also experienced bouts of severe abdominal bloating, cramping, and constipation.

In the previous year, she had experienced four sinus infections and was plagued by recurrent sinus headaches. Although she had no history of allergies, she was now having wheezing attacks and allergic reactions to perfumes, hairsprays, smoke, and a variety of chemical fumes.

On top of all this, Maggie suffered from severe depression and fatigue. She complained that she was in a "brain fog" much of the time.

Maggie had sought the care of a number of physicians in her hometown of St. Louis, Missouri. She had been given antibiotics for her sinus infections, which had made her abdominal bloating worse, and antidepressants for her mood problems, which had provided no relief. When a friend of hers, who was a patient at the Hotze Health & Wellness Center, told her there was a natural alternative treatment for her problems, Maggie flew to Houston for an evaluation.

After telling me of her numerous problems, Maggie asked, "Dr. Hotze, am I a hypochondriac?"

WHY DOCTORS DON'T UNDERSTAND WOMEN

The physicians Maggie consulted made her feel as if her problems were all in her head. As you will see, they were wrong. Although their attitudes to Maggie's complaints were condescending, they were not surprising. If their medical education was anything like mine, then a callous disregard for women's health problems was virtually guaranteed. Let me explain.

During my first semester of medical school, I took a course called History and Physical Diagnosis. This is a basic course in which medical students learn to interview a patient, identify the chief complaint or symptom, and then perform a review of the systems (digestive, respiratory, cardiovascular, musculoskeletal, etc.), asking about other symptoms the patient might be having.

The professor teaching this course instructed us that if a woman in midlife had more than one complaint during the review of systems, then she was a hypochondriac and should be placed on an antidepressant.

Now, imagine this. The class was overwhelmingly comprised of young men in their early twenties. Every man in that room had already experienced numerous problems with a girlfriend or spouse. Now they knew why. The professor was asserting that women were emotionally unstable individuals, so much so that they often needed antidepressants to make them tolerable. This was a small seed that was sown in the minds of all those young, would-be doctors. It was a seed that would sprout years later when they finally began their own medical practices. The first time they had to interview a middle-aged female patient, she would typically describe a long list of complaints. "Voila," they would think. The professor had been right about women. And of course they knew exactly what to do: prescribe an antidepressant.

What a sad commentary this is. The vast majority of women who have come to me for evaluations are already taking antidepressants, which are one of the most widely prescribed classes of drugs. Now you know why.

Maggie's Story: "I Feel Like I'm Falling Apart"

When Maggie and I sat down for our first meeting, I asked her how she was feeling.

"I feel like I'm falling apart," she said. "I expected motherhood to be a time of enjoyment and excitement, but instead I feel sad and cry all the time. It is difficult for me to sleep and I never feel fully rested. I can't focus, I have no desire for sex, and I'm not the mother or the wife I want to be."

"How has this affected your relationship with your husband?" I asked.

"He doesn't understand what is going on with me. At first he tried to be supportive but then he became totally exasperated. So I did what most women do. I went to see my doctor."

I asked Maggie what her doctor had done to help her.

"My doctor said that I was depressed and sent me to a psychiatrist, who put me on antidepressants. They both made me feel like I was a hypochondriac. When the antidepressants didn't work, I was scared they might be right. But deep down, I know I'm not crazy and that something isn't right in my body. I can't imagine living this way the rest of my life."

I reassured Maggie that she didn't have to live this way. I told her that there was a simple explanation for her symptoms and a simple solution to her health problems.

ESTROGEN DOMINANCE AFTER PREGNANCY

During pregnancy, the baby's placenta produces high levels of progesterone—ten to twenty times higher than a woman normally produces. When the baby is delivered and the placenta expelled, there is a precipitous drop in progesterone levels. However, estrogen levels remain very high. Unless the ovaries can produce adequate amounts of progesterone to balance the estrogen, a condition known as estrogen dominance will occur.

Childbirth is not the only cause of estrogen dominance. It can also occur at puberty, after discontinuing birth control pills, after tubal ligation or hysterectomy, or simply as a woman moves through her menstrual life. Imbalances in the levels of estrogen and progesterone are inevitable for women in their thirties, forties, and beyond. Regardless of the cause of this imbalance, the health problems that arise are often severe and debilitating. For Maggie, the dramatic change in her hormonal balance following the birth of her child stressed her adrenal glands, altered her thyroid function, and triggered her allergic disorders.

Maggie's Treatment Program

I reassured Maggie that her symptoms were common to women in her age group and could be easily treated. We started by addressing the imbalance in her female hormone levels. Since Maggie was producing adequate estrogen, boosting her progesterone levels would be the key to restoring proper hormonal balance. This could be accomplished safely with a natural, biologically identical progesterone supplement to be taken on days fifteen through twenty-eight of her menstrual cycle.

Maggie's history indicated that she was suffering from low thyroid function, so I prescribed natural thyroid hormone, Armour Thyroid, to correct this deficit. Because Maggie's hormonal imbalance had stressed her adrenal glands, I also advised her to take a small dose of the natural adrenal hormone, cortisol.

Maggie's recurrent sinus infections are a classic feature of allergies. Skin testing enabled me to determine the level at which to start her allergy treatment for common airborne allergies. Rather than giving Maggie a series of shots to desensitize her to allergens, I prescribed sublingual (under-the-tongue) allergy drops. I explained to her that this innovative approach to the treatment of allergies is safe, convenient, and very effective.

Maggie was weaned off antidepressants, which were replaced with a natural mood-elevating compound, 5-HTP. This molecule is the precursor to serotonin, a neurotransmitter that plays a key role in regulating both mood and sleep. Maggie started a customized program of nutritional supplements and a nutritionally balanced eating program.

Because Maggie's antibiotic use had contributed to yeast overgrowth and digestive problems, I explained that it was important for her to remain on a yeast-free diet for at least three months in order to restore health to her digestive tract. She was prescribed medication to kill yeast, along with preparations of Lactobacillus acidophilus to replenish beneficial bacteria in the colon that are so important to intestinal health.

Maggie responded beautifully to this comprehensive treatment program. Within one month of beginning treatment, her depression and fatigue had resolved and her menstrual cycle had normalized. She was sleeping well and feeling rested upon awakening. Her energy was so much better that she even began a daily jogging program.

Two years later, Maggie gave birth to her second child. Because her hormones were balanced, she bounced back quickly and had none of the postpartum problems that she had experienced after her first pregnancy. When she returned to the office recently for follow-up, she told me, "I feel healthy, energetic, and happy. Thank you for giving me back my life."

A ROAD MAP TO RECOVERY

Women like Maggie are seen at the Hotze Health & Wellness Center every day. Many travel from out of state, and most have already been evaluated by several doctors before we see them. They have been prescribed numerous drugs to treat their hormonal imbalances, menstrual irregularities, depression, allergies, infections, and other health problems. Yet, despite the fact that they have been given "the best that medicine has to offer," they feel no better than they did before they took the drugs prescribed to them. In fact, they often feel worse.

This is no surprise to me. The simple fact is that, with few exceptions, prescription drugs are not cures, nor are they intended to be. By and large, prescription drugs are designed to relieve symptoms. But just as putting a new coat of paint on a house won't fix a cracked foundation, prescribing a drug to alleviate a patient's symptoms will not restore the patient to good health. It's no wonder many women who come to me tell me they feel like they are falling apart.

In the next chapter, I will tell you more about how and why I stopped practicing drug-based medicine and began to explore safe and effective alternatives to help my patients restore their health. As you will see, I didn't venture off the beaten path without a struggle. After all, I had been inculcated with the belief that practicing medicine was virtually synonymous with prescribing drugs. The truth is, I left mainstream medicine reluctantly and only after a series of events in my personal and professional life convinced me that there was a better way, a more natural way, to help my patients regain their health and vitality. Once I began to witness the amazing recoveries of my patients as they implemented these natural therapies, there was no turning back.

This book is a road map that will guide you to the path of health and wellness that thousands of my patients have traveled. It is a map that you can use in your own quest for good health, abundant energy, and the joy that comes from living life to the fullest.

CHAPTER 3
Challenging Herd Mentality

My father, Ernest Hotze, was an engineer who rose to become vice president of sales for Dresser Clark. He later went on to establish his own business, Compressor Engineering Corporation (CECO). Dad was an outstanding salesman and entrepreneur. With seven sons and one daughter, he had to be. Dad instilled in us a desire to excel beyond the norm and hold ourselves to high standards.

My mother, Margaret, who earned a journalism degree from the University of Texas, was a voracious reader. She constantly challenged us to "break out of the box" and question conventional thought. If she told us once, she told us a hundred times, "Never follow the crowd because it is usually going in the wrong direction. Move away from the crowd and lead it in the right direction."

During my years at St. Thomas High School, an all-boys' school in Houston, I took her leadership advice to heart. I ran for and was elected student body president. I also played quarterback for the football team. Nothing was more exhilarating to me than getting into a tight situation, pulling the team together in a huddle, and calling the play.

The football coaches at St. Thomas reinforced the values that I had received at home, challenging us to excel. Though we played many of the top-ranked public high schools, every time we set foot on the field we fully expected to win. And win we did. We played in the Texas Catholic Interscholastic State Championship every year I was in high school, and we won the state title three out of four years.

The winning spirit instilled in me by my parents and my coaches has produced a steel-willed determination to overcome obstacles as I seek to achieve my goals. My experiences have taught me that with every adversity there is a seed of equal or greater opportunity in the future.

Football also brought my wife of thirty-six years into my life. Janie, who attended Duchesne Academy, an all-girls' school, was one of our varsity cheerleaders. During the summer after our senior year in high school, Janie and I eloped to Mexico. I do not think this is what my mother had in mind when she advised me not to follow the crowd. My father told me that I had made my bed and I was going to have to sleep in it. With seven other children, he was in no position to help us financially, nor did we expect that of him.

Janie and I moved to Austin, Texas, so that I could attend college. Janie worked for the first few years of our marriage, until the birth of our second child, while I attended the University of Texas and set up a paint contracting and remodeling business. Even though I was working, I managed to graduate from college in three and a half years. Little did I know it, but my real education was only about to begin: I was going to medical school.

A CULTURE OF CONFORMITY

In 1972, I entered the University of Texas Medical School at Houston. The first two years consisted solely of classroom lectures and laboratory work. The final two years were clinical rotations in internal medicine, obstetrics and gynecology, psychiatry, pediatrics, cardiology, surgery, and other specialties.

Medical school required some adjustment. After years of thinking outside the box, I found myself in an environment where questioning the status quo was not encouraged. The young doctors-to-be were expected to receive instruction from their elders, not question it. This didn't come naturally to me.

My psychiatry rotation proved to be my most difficult. Most of the patients in the psychiatric wards of the hospital were taking mind-altering medications such as antidepressants, antipsychotics, lithium, and tranquilizers. Their faces were expressionless, with emptiness in their eyes. They walked in a jerky manner and made rolling motions with their fingers. These were the side effects of the powerful drugs that they had been prescribed.

I also observed patients with depression undergoing electroshock therapy. The doctor would place paddles on each side of the patient's head and administer currents of electricity. When the patients were shocked, their bodies would become rigid and undergo seizurelike activity. Because the electric shock to the brain would destroy memory, patients often remained depressed after this therapy but did not remember why. The treatment was barbaric.

During my psychiatric rotation, I read a book called *The Myth of Mental Illness*, by Dr. Tom Szasz, a prominent psychiatrist. In this book, he criticized what he called the "psycho-babble" of modern-day psychiatry and its attempt to redefine psychological problems as medical diseases. By classifying peculiarities of thinking or behavior as diseases, he charged, psychiatry had absolved individuals of responsibility for their actions. The drug companies capitalized on this by synthesizing a host of medications to "treat" these new diseases.

Dr. Szasz's arguments impressed me. Unfortunately, my professors did not share my point of view and gave me an F at the end of my psychiatry rotation. I was required to retake psychiatry the spring of my fourth year in medical school. Since passing this clinical rotation was a requirement of graduation, I decided that discretion was the better part of valor. So the second time around, I spouted back exactly what my psychiatry professors wanted to hear and earned a passing grade.

It was during my surgical rotation that I was taught the surgeons' motto: "A chance to cut is a chance to cure." The surgeons I encountered tended to frown upon the use of drugs, recognizing—quite rightly—that drugs do not cure disease but merely alleviate symptoms. However, they simply replaced one technique for managing symptoms with a more extreme one: cutting or removing the organ in which the symptoms were manifested.

During my surgical rotation, I witnessed this drastic approach to symptom management countless times. For example, hysterectomies were routinely recommended when women experienced heavy menstrual bleeding and cramps. The surgeons performing these operations believed that removing the target organ, the uterus, would cure the problem. Well, yes, without a uterus a woman will no longer experience heavy periods and breakthrough bleeding. But what if the uterus was not the cause of the problem? More important, what if the underlying cause could be identified and corrected? If this was possible, millions of women could be spared the ordeal of surgery and the host of problems resulting from removal of the uterus and ovaries.

These were not questions I felt prepared to ask at this early stage in my medical career. But soon enough I would meet a mentor who would encourage me to ask them.

LEARNING TO ASK WHY

In 1976, I graduated from medical school, passed the state boards, and received my medical license. That fall, I began my surgical internship at St. Joseph's Hospital in Houston.

During my internship I was fortunate to work under a remarkable physician, Herb Fred, M.D. Dr. Fred was the director of postgraduate education at St. Joseph's Hospital. He was a brilliant clinician who was able to see the big picture. He taught the newly minted M.D.s the necessity of making our diagnoses based upon the clinical history and physical examination of our patients, rather than by relying upon laboratory tests.

Dr. Fred used the Socratic method of teaching. When we presented patient cases with our diagnoses to Dr. Fred, he would always ask us, "Why is that so?" We would respond, and he would again ask, "Well, why is that so?" This dialogue would continue until he had exposed our ignorance and demonstrated that, in fact, we did not know why it was so.

Dr. Fred was emphatic in his message that we would never become excellent physicians unless we learned to ask why. Why does this patient have recurrent infections? Why does this patient have headaches? Why is this patient fatigued or depressed? In short, what is the underlying cause of this patient's symptoms? And as a corollary to that, why should I believe that drugs, with their numerous side effects, will resolve this patient's problems? Could there be a safer, more natural way to address the underlying cause?

Unfortunately, there are not many professors like Dr. Fred who challenge their students to question conventional thinking. The implicit message I received during most of my medical education was that poor health was inevitable—and that, when it occurred, the solution was a prescription drug.

A BITTER PILL TO SWALLOW

After completing my postgraduate training, I practiced emergency medicine for five years. Then, in 1981, I opened my own medical practice in Houston. For the first six years or so, I practiced medicine as I had been taught, prescribing drugs to palliate my patients' symptoms. When one drug caused a side effect, I would simply prescribe another to address the new problem.

Not surprisingly, the patients did not get better with this approach. When I treated my patients' upper respiratory infections with an antibiotic, it seemed that many would return within a relatively short period of time with another infection. I found myself flinching when I asked my patients how they were doing, expecting the common answer, "I still don't feel well."

One day, a patient who lived in a retirement home near my office came in for a follow-up evaluation. Of course, the first thing I asked her was, "How are you doing, Mrs. Jones?" She stated, "Dr. Hotze, ever since I threw away all of the medications you were giving me, I feel like a million dollars!" Her remark hit me like a ton of bricks. This patient was wise because she recognized that the drugs that I had prescribed for her made her feel worse than she had felt prior to taking them. The old adage had proven true, "The cure is often worse than the disease."

If there was ever any doubt that she was right, then my father's experience drove this lesson home to me. Dad, who at seventy was being treated for high blood pressure but was still CEO of Compressor Engineering Corporation, had been preaching to me that the secret to good health was an afternoon nap.

One day, Dad dropped by my office and asked me to check his blood pressure. He revealed that his doctor, a prominent Houston cardiologist, had prescribed Inderal. This drug was the first of a class of antihypertensive drugs called beta blockers, and I knew that it had a lengthy list of side effects, including fatigue, depression, mental confusion, and impotence.

When my father told me he was using Inderal, I said, "Dad, no wonder you have to take a nap every afternoon. That drug may lower your blood pressure but it also causes fatigue and other side effects. Let me put you on a newer, safer blood pressure medication and see if you don't feel better." Two days later, my father called me at my office to tell me that he felt two thousand percent better—not one hundred or two hundred percent, but two thousand percent better.

Not long after that, my brother Bruce, who was the president of my father's corporation, contacted me and asked, "What the heck are you giving Dad?"

"Why do you ask?"

"He's storming around the office, taking charge of everything," Bruce replied.

"Is he still taking afternoon naps?"

"No."

"All I did was change his blood pressure medication. He was on Inderal, which causes severe mental and physical tiredness. Now that he's stopped Inderal and is on a newer, safer medication, he has regained his energy."

A few weeks later, my father gave me a copy of a letter that he had sent to his cardiologist, summarily firing him. In the letter, he asked the cardiologist how many other men had been prescribed this drug and experienced fatigue, depression, and impotence. Dad stated in his letter that Inderal should be banned.

A SURGICAL CATASTROPHE

In 1988, my father came by my office and told me that he had been experiencing chest pain. After examining him, I recommended that he let my brother drive him to the hospital to be evaluated by a cardiologist. Dad was hospitalized and underwent cardiac catheterization, a diagnostic procedure to evaluate the integrity of the heart and coronary arteries.

Blood tests and an electrocardiogram had shown no evidence of a heart attack. However, during the catheterization, the cardiologist noted that my father had a blockage in one of his coronary arteries. He immediately performed angioplasty, a procedure in which a balloon is guided through the catheter to the blockage and then inflated. This is supposed to press the blockage against the artery walls, widening the artery and improving blood flow. After the procedure, my father's chest pain was resolved and he was discharged from the hospital.

Three months later, my father's chest pain returned and he was readmitted to the hospital. His cardiologist performed a repeat angioplasty the following day. I was outside the cardiac catheterization lab watching the procedure through a glass window and monitoring my father's electrocardiogram on the computer screen. Suddenly, there was a dramatic change in the wave pattern, indicating a loss of blood flow to a major portion of my father's heart. I knew that a disaster had occurred. In the attempt to expand my father's left anterior descending coronary artery, which is the main artery of the heart, the artery had ruptured.

Immediately, I contacted Dr. Robert Feldtman, a cardiovascular surgeon and close friend of the family who was on standby in case a complication developed. My father was rushed to the operating room for emergency cardiac bypass surgery. Dad was seventy-two years of age at this time. He was still managing a manufacturing business with over 175 employees and running two miles every day, as he had done for nearly twenty years. He was in excellent shape for his age and this allowed him to survive the surgery. Unfortunately, he had suffered irreparable damage to his heart, which eventually enlarged to the size of a football.

Two weeks after Dad's surgery, I was visiting him at home and he said, "I don't know what in the world I was thinking, letting the doctor try to dilate my coronary artery. Because my artery was already calcified, there was no way it could be dilated without shattering the arterial wall." My dad was speaking from his engineering background.

A Prayer . . . and an Answer

By the time of my father's surgical catastrophe, I had been a doctor for thirteen years, and in private practice for the previous seven years. I had entered medicine hoping to heal people, and yet, by and large, this wasn't happening. My patients were telling me that they felt better without the drugs I gave them. My father had pointed out to me a fundamental flaw in the angioplasty procedure—and had paid dearly for it. All the seemingly solid truths that had been handed down to me in medical school now seemed as flimsy as tissue paper.

I was thirty-nine, happily married to a devoted wife, the proud father of eight children. And yet I felt discouraged by the thought of continuing in a vocation that was no longer fulfilling. I knew that if I was going to make a change, it had to be now. I shared my disenchantment with my wife, Janie. We prayed together, asking God to help me find a way to help my patients get well and feel well, and at the same time be able to earn enough to raise my family and provide them with the same opportunities that our parents had provided us.

My prayers were answered as they so often were—in a form that was both an opportunity and a challenge.

CHAPTER 4

Encounter with an Allergist

In January 1989, a general surgeon and my close friend, Dr. Stephen McElmurry, contacted me about relocating my office to the rapidly growing West Houston/Katy area. Steve introduced me to Warren Willke, the hospital administrator of Katy Medical Center. Warren informed me that an office would be available soon in his building and invited me to come out and take a look at it.

As it turned out, the physician who was moving out of the space was an allergist by the name of Dr. David Ziegler. When I visited the location, I had the opportunity to meet with him. Looking back, it was a providential encounter. While I was discouraged with my conventional medical practice, Dr. Ziegler described his practice of allergy medicine as enjoyable and satisfying. He told me of his ability to help his patients get well, and he had plenty of case histories to support his assertion.

"Why don't you incorporate the treatment of allergies into your medical practice," he suggested, "and see for yourself what a difference it will make in your patients' lives?"

I turned that question over in my mind, recalling my own experience with severe childhood allergies. As a young boy whose deep chest cough was so loud that it could be heard throughout St. Michael's Grade School, I had been evaluated for everything from cancer to tuberculosis at the Houston Diagnostic Center. When the doctors there were unable to identify the cause of my coughing, my mother finally took me to an allergist. After I was tested, I began allergy desensitization injections, which I administered to myself every week at home for five years.

Unfortunately, my medical school education had included only an hour on the subject of allergies. "How can I begin to gain the necessary knowledge that would allow me to incorporate the treatment of allergies into my medical practice?" I asked Dr. Ziegler.

Dr. Ziegler told me about a medical society called the Pan American Allergy Society that trained physicians to treat allergic disorders—and their annual meeting would be taking place the very next month in San Antonio. So I decided to attend.

AN INFUSION OF HOPE

At the Pan American Allergy Society conference, I listened to lectures by physicians who used the same method of evaluating patients as did my earlier mentor, Dr. Herb Fred. When they saw patients with seemingly intractable health problems, they did not assume that these problems were caused by a lack of prescription drugs. Instead, they persistently asked why. Why is this patient having recurrent infections? Why does this patient get headaches on a regular basis? Why does this patient have eczema?

The lecturers presented numerous case studies of patients with problems ranging from sinus infections and skin disorders to asthma and migraine headaches. These patients' chronic health problems finally began to improve when their allergies were identified and treated. It could have been any number of my patients whom the speakers were presenting during the conference lectures—only these patients were actually improving. To a physician who had almost given up hope of helping his patients feel better, this was exciting news.

The caliber of the lectures at this conference and the enthusiasm of the physicians for helping their patients get well naturally made a strong and positive impression on me. Before the conference ended, I was certain that this was a path I wanted to follow.

After his lecture, I approached Dr. James Willoughby, who was then president of the Pan American Allergy Society. "Dr. Willoughby," I said, "I want to practice medicine just the way you do."

"Then come up to my office in Kansas City and let me train you," he replied.

Over the next few months, I made several trips to Dr. Willoughby's office in Kansas City, where he taught me his techniques for treating patients with allergic disorders. Dr. Willoughby's son Tom, who managed Antigen Laboratories, and his daughter-in-law Betsy, who was one of his nurses, were instrumental in helping me set up my allergy practice, which I opened in July 1989.

Initially, with only one person on my staff, I performed all the skin testing and prepared and administered all the allergy injections. To my delight, my patients started to get well! This was very encouraging to me and to them. There was hope!

With a burning desire to learn more about natural approaches to medical problems, I joined the American Academy of Environmental Medicine. I took the examination for the American Academy of Otolaryngic Allergy and was certified as a Fellow Member of this organization. I attended every possible continuing education conference relating to allergies.

By the fall of 1991, the steady growth of my medical practice led me to purchase an office building in the West Houston area to expand my facilities. In that same year I was invited to join the board of directors of the Pan American Allergy Society.

Thus began my career as an allergist.

WHAT IS AN ALLERGY?

An allergy is an abnormal reaction by the body's immune system to normally occurring substances that cause no problem for most people. Common environmental allergens include weed, tree, and grass pollens; dust mites; mold spores; and animal dander. Common foods such as wheat, corn, eggs, milk, yeast, or soybeans also may cause allergic reactions. In most children with eczema, the cause is a food allergy. Recurrent ear infections in children are caused by a milk allergy in at least 50 percent of cases. You may know someone who gets a headache after drinking wine or develops hives after eating shellfish or peanuts. These are all examples of food allergies.

If you've ever set off a car alarm accidentally by brushing past an automobile in a parking lot, you know how disturbing an experience that can be. An encounter with a substance to which you are allergic causes a similar response by your body's "alarm system."

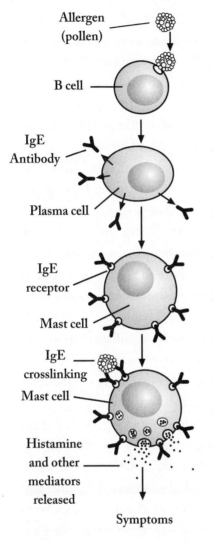

The first time an allergen enters the body and binds to a B cell, the cell is stimulated to mature into an antibody-producing "factory" called a plasma cell.

The plasma cell churns out IgE antibodies specific to the allergen, which attach to specialized receptors on mast cells, priming them for subsequent encounters.

The next time the allergen enters the body, it binds to and crosslinks with IgE antibodies, causing the mast cell to release histamine and other powerful chemicals that trigger allergy symptoms.

Figure 1. The allergic response.

This is how you become sensitized "allergic" to a substance. The first time an allergen such as ragweed pollen or wheat enters the body, the immune system makes antibodies specific to the allergen. These antibodies then attach themselves to mast cells, specialized white blood cells that cover the lining of the mucous membranes of the respiratory and digestive tracts. The binding of these antibodies to the mast cells sensitizes them to the allergen so that they are primed to react at the next exposure to it.

The next time the allergen enters the body, the mast cells release massive quantities of histamine and other inflammatory chemicals in an attempt to get rid of the offending substance. These chemicals cause blood vessels to dilate, prompting tissue swelling, tearing of the eyes, and nasal discharge. They also stimulate secretion of large amounts of mucus and cause the bronchial tubes to constrict, triggering coughing and wheezing.

Although respiratory discomfort is the most obvious indicator of an allergic reaction, allergies can cause symptoms throughout the body depending on where the immune system is activated. Food allergens can trigger gastrointestinal symptoms such as canker sores, gastritis, and diarrhea. Headaches, depression, anxiety, and memory problems can occur if inflammation and swelling affect the brain. Recurrent or chronic urinary tract infections, childhood ear infections, upper respiratory infections, and yeast infections commonly have an allergic basis.

Childhood asthma is due to underlying allergies. The most common offenders are dust mites, which live by the millions in bedding and pillows, and foods such as wheat, corn, eggs, milk, yeast, and soybeans. Adult asthma is caused by allergies as well. Other serious conditions, including rheumatoid arthritis and irritable bowel syndrome, can be exacerbated by allergies, especially allergies to foods.

Common Allergy Symptoms:
- Fatigue
- Frequent headaches
- Sneezing, postnasal drainage or itching of the nose
- Frequent "colds"
- Recurrent or chronic sinus infections

- Recurrent yeast infections, jock itch, or athlete's foot
- Dizziness
- Itching, watering, redness, or swelling of the eyes
- Dark circles under the eyes
- Recurrent ear infections
- Recurrent cough or bronchitis
- Tightness in the chest, wheezing, or asthma
- Eczema, skin rashes, itching, or hives
- Indigestion, bloating, diarrhea, or constipation

WHO GETS ALLERGIES?

At least 40 percent of Americans suffer from allergies, and the number is growing. Without a doubt, there is a genetic basis to allergies. Children are more likely to develop allergies if one or more parents is allergic. Although childhood is the time when many allergies first become apparent, this is more often true for males than females. In reality, allergies can emerge at any age and are especially likely to develop during times of stress, when the body's defenses are lowered, such as after a viral infection, during puberty, during or after pregnancy, after a severe injury, or following emotional loss.

Remember Maggie, the young woman I wrote about in chapter 2? Although Maggie had no history of allergies, after the birth of her first child she began having recurrent sinus infections and sinus headaches, wheezing attacks, fatigue, and digestive problems. None of the doctors she consulted had diagnosed her allergic condition, even though Maggie's symptoms were all red flags for allergy.

In my practice, I often see women of Maggie's age or older who suddenly begin experiencing allergies and recurrent upper respiratory infections. As in Maggie's case, these symptoms may occur after childbirth. They may also be associated with a change in menstrual cycles, tubal ligation, hysterectomy, or menopause. Many people are not aware that allergies can occur at any age, including midlife. Unless these allergies are identified and treated, chronic health problems can result. Consider the following questions to evaluate the likelihood that you suffer from allergies.

- Do your symptoms worsen during a particular season, such as the spring or fall?
- Are your symptoms worse in parks or grassy areas?
- Are your symptoms worse around animals?
- Do your symptoms change when you go indoors or outdoors?
- Are your symptoms worse when you come into contact with dust?
- Are your symptoms worse upon arising in the morning?
- Do you awaken in the middle of the night with congestion?
- Do you have mood swings or feel depressed for no particular reason?
- Do you develop symptoms after eating or drinking certain foods?
- Do you sometimes feel stimulated, hyperactive, or fatigued after meals?
- Do you have any blood relatives with allergies?

ALLERGY DRUGS MASK SYMPTOMS

Many allergy patients whom I have evaluated have been "managing" their illness with antihistamines. These drugs do not prevent the mast cells from releasing histamine, but they do decrease histamine's ability to cause reactions in the respiratory tract and elsewhere. Because histamine and other inflammatory chemicals are to blame for the runny nose, watery eyes, scratchy throat, mucus, and bronchial constriction that accompany allergies, antihistamines may provide a measure of relief.

However, like antidepressants, antispasmodics, and other drugs with "anti" in their names, antihistamines do not correct the underlying problem. Keep in mind that allergies are caused by an overreactive immune system that misidentifies harmless substances as threatening invaders. Nowhere on the label of an antihistamine will you see information that this drug helps retrain the immune system to stop overreacting to allergens. What you will see, though, is a list of side effects that the antihistamine can cause, such as fatigue, drowsiness, dry mouth, loss of appetite, stomach upset, nausea, blurred vision, dizziness, headaches, and skin rashes.

Many over-the-counter antihistamines interfere with histamine receptors in the brain. Because your brain uses naturally occurring histamine to maintain alertness, these drugs are notorious for causing drowsiness and mental impairment. In fact, one over-the-counter antihistamine, diphenhydramine (Benadryl), is so effective at inducing drowsiness that it is also sold as a sleep aid!

A Doctor's Finest Instruments

In this era of high-tech medicine, many physicians are more interested in ordering laboratory tests than they are in listening to the history and the symptoms of their patients. However, a lab test is at best a snapshot in time and provides only limited information about a patient's health status. Patients provide a tremendous amount of crucial information through their history and symptoms, but this information is of value only if the physician takes time to listen. The physician must then fit together the pieces of the puzzle using the finest instruments God has given him: his ears, eyes, and brain.

A lot of information about the likelihood of allergies can be discovered simply by listening to and looking at a patient. A crease across the bridge of the nose, watery or puffy eyes, dark circles under the eyes, skin rashes or blotches, nasal congestion, and coughing or wheezing are all physical signs that may indicate an allergy. In my practice, a lengthy interview precedes every patient's appointment and provides information that is crucial to diagnosing allergies. This interview covers the patient's family history, their personal history of illness, and their present symptoms. Unlike the "snapshot" provided by a lab test, this interview gives me a three-dimensional time-lapsed view of each patient's health status.

An allergy skin test is administered to a patient only after I have made the diagnosis of an allergic disorder based upon my comprehensive history and physical examination. The technique I use is the highly accurate skin test called serial endpoint titration (SET). SET involves administering a series of dilutions of suspected allergens beneath the skin and observing the response.

This series of skin tests is used not only to identify the offending allergen but also to determine the proper dose of the allergen with which to begin treatment—a dose that is strong enough to rally the immune system to produce allergy-blocking antibodies but not so strong as to cause a full-blown allergic reaction.

Allergy treatment is known as desensitization. The goal is to decrease or eliminate the immune system's reaction to offending allergens that are causing symptoms. Desensitization treatment works according to the principle, "Fight fire with fire." By administering a weak dilution of the very allergens to which the patient is allergic, the patient's immune system is reeducated. New "blocking" antibodies are produced that reduce the immune system's reactivity to the offending substances. Gradually, the patient receives increasingly more concentrated dilutions of the allergen until a plateau is reached where the patient is no longer reactive to the substance.

This is the technique that I learned from Dr. James Willoughby, and it is the technique that I use today—with one slight, but very significant change.

Shots Are Out. Drops Are In.

That's right! There is no longer a need to get allergy shots because you can now take allergy desensitization treatment sublingually (under the tongue). Who enjoys getting allergy shots, anyway? Not only do you have to drive to the doctor's office for the weekly allergy injection, but also you have to wait before you receive your shot, and then wait after your shot to make sure you do not have an adverse reaction. Sublingually administered allergy drops are safe, effective allergy desensitization treatments that are widely used in Europe. In fact, they are the only method used in Great Britain. The World Health Organization (WHO) recognizes allergy drops as a viable alternative to injections.

In September of 1996, John, a good friend from high school, called me to complain about his asthma. John owns a car dealership and loves to hunt deer and quail. But this presents him with a problem every year because hunting season is in the fall, and fall is weed pollen season in Texas. This is when John develops his asthma. His eyes itch, get watery, and swell. His nasal passages get congested and he starts coughing and wheezing.

John had been evaluated at my office in 1994 and started on allergy shots. However, because of the difficulty of traveling to my office each week for his injection, he was inconsistent in his treatment. The only time he got serious about taking his allergy shots was during the fall allergy season. By then, it was too late for the treatment to be effective.

In the fall of 1996, I told John that I was going to start him on allergy desensitization drops instead of shots as a way to manage his allergies and asthma. This is the same treatment that I had been prescribing for children since 1989, and it had been working well. Many of my allergy colleagues from around the country had been praising the benefits of using allergy drops to treat allergic disorders in all patients, but I had resisted because I was convinced that injections were superior to the drops.

When John came to see me, I said, "I don't know how these are going to work, but you are a whole lot better getting allergy treatment by drops than not at all." I instructed him to take one allergy drop under his tongue daily.

The next time I ran into John was over the Christmas holidays of that same year, at which time he told me that the drops I gave him for his allergies were "magic drops." He had no asthma problems at all that fall, and he continued taking the drops from then on.

At that point, I became a believer in the effectiveness of treating allergic disorders using allergy drops. The drops contain identical allergens as in allergy injections, except in a more concentrated form. Taking a drop daily is equivalent to having an injection weekly. My patients could now save time by taking their allergy treatments at home, without having to travel and wait at my office.

Allergy drops are much safer and, in my clinical judgment, much more effective than the allergy injections. This may be due to the simple fact that the patients are more compliant in taking their treatment. In the fifteen years that I have been prescribing them, we have never had a significant adverse reaction to the allergy drops in the more than four thousand patients who have used them.

Unfortunately, most allergists in America are far less open-minded about using allergy drops than their European counterparts. Trying to find a physician in this country who offers allergy drops as an alternative to shots is difficult. The reason for this is that most insurance companies will not routinely cover allergy drop treatment. Who do you think this benefits, the allergy patients or the insurance companies?

For more information about sublingual allergy drops, visit www.allergychoices.com. Allergy Choices, located in La Crosse, Wisconsin, was founded by David L. Morris, M.D., who is a fellow in the American College of Allergists. Dr. Morris began publishing papers in the medical literature on sublingual immunotherapy in 1969 and became board certified by the American Board of Allergy and Immunology in 1974. He is recognized as a leading authority on the subject of sublingual immunotherapy.

CROSS REACTIONS

If you suffer from an airborne allergy, certain foods can exacerbate your symptoms by altering your body's response to the allergen. To minimize the likelihood of a cross reaction, these foods should be avoided during the season in which the airborne allergen is present.

Airborne allergen	Foods to avoid
Grass (March-September)	Legumes (beans and peas)
Ragweed (August-December)	Eggs, milk, mint
Pigweed (March-December)	Pork, black peppers
Sage (August-December)	Potatoes, tomatoes
Mesquite (April-December)	Cane sugar, oranges
Dust (Year-round)	Oysters
Molds (Year-round)	Cheese, mushrooms

TREATMENT OF FOOD ALLERGIES

As with airborne allergies, food allergies can be identified using skin testing. At my office, we test for thirty-five of the most common food allergens, including wheat, corn, eggs, milk, yeast, and soybeans. We also recommend oral challenge testing for further determination of food allergy.

The purpose of the oral challenge test is to determine if symptoms will result after eating a suspected allergenic food.

The suspected food is included in the diet for four days, then eliminated for four days. On the ninth day, in the morning, the suspected food is eaten alone with a glass of pure water. After eating the food, the patient monitors the development of new symptoms during the first hour. If no symptoms develop, a second portion of the food is eaten and the patient continues to watch for immediate and delayed symptoms for the next forty-eight hours. The symptoms may be any one of the allergy symptoms previously listed. If no symptoms occur, then the food can be safely added back into the diet.

If symptoms develop when a food is introduced, then this food is likely to be allergenic. As with airborne allergens, we use sublingual neutralization drops to desensitize the immune system to the food. Over time, this may allow the patient to reintroduce the food into the diet on a rotated basis, every four days.

The elimination/rotation diet is another approach to identifying and managing food allergies. The patient starts with a one-month low-allergenic diet. The following foods may be eaten, unless the patient has had a skin reaction to them: chicken, turkey, beef, pork, fish, lamb, fresh vegetables, beans, rice, potatoes, and salads with cold-pressed olive oil. This diet is followed for one month. Then every two days, one new food is introduced in its purest form, and any symptoms that arise are noted.

If symptoms arise, indicating an allergy, sublingual allergy drops can be prescribed to help neutralize the symptoms. On the other hand, if no symptoms appear, this food probably can be added back into the diet, rotating it every fourth day. Food allergies often arise from eating the same foods day after day, and a diversified rotation diet is the best way to avoid developing new food allergies. This type of diet involves eating foods from a different "family" each day for four days, then beginning the cycle again. (See appendix D for more information.)

Did You Know That . . .

- Up to 75 percent of asthmatics have an undiagnosed food allergy.
- It is possible to become "addicted" to an allergenic food. Eating the allergenic food may bring short-term relief of symptoms but causes chronic symptoms.
- Roughly 90 percent of food allergies are caused by just a few foods: wheat, corn, milk, eggs, yeast, soybean, peanuts, nuts, fish, and shellfish.
- Food allergies may cause a flare-up of symptoms within an hour after eating, in the late afternoon, or in the early morning hours (1–5 a.m.).
- Itching between the shoulder blades may be a referred sensation from the esophagus and trachea, indicating a food allergy.
- Dehydration can worsen allergy symptoms by prompting the release of histamine. Drinking plenty of water helps minimize the release of histamine.
- The most common complaint of allergy is fatigue.

A Patient Success Story

Since entering the practice of allergy medicine in 1989, I have helped thousands of patients recover from allergies and regain their energy and health. But perhaps no story is more dramatic than that of Bob, a lifelong asthmatic who suffered a nearly fatal reaction to an over-the-counter antihistamine when he was in his thirties. Bob's heart stopped several times in the hospital emergency room and had to be restarted with a defibrillator. Fortunately, Bob survived this ordeal and suffered no permanent damage to his heart.

Bob's doctor monitored his condition closely for the next two years, prescribing numerous drugs to treat his asthma, allergies, and sinus infections. Not surprisingly, Bob didn't get better using these drugs. In fact, he got worse. In one year, he was on antibiotics for seven months for treatment of his chronic sinus infections.

Finally, Bob's doctor admitted defeat and insisted that Bob consult an ear, nose, and throat surgeon. After all, "a chance to cut is a chance to cure." Bob underwent surgery twice to repair his sinuses and achieved some relief from his asthma. But even after two surgeries, he was still taking steroids, using an inhaler, and having severe asthma attacks that sent him to the emergency room. When one drug didn't work, his doctor would prescribe another. After an inhaler caused Bob's blood pressure to soar, his doctor prescribed an antihypertensive drug.

Bob realized that prescribing one drug to correct the symptoms caused by another was not a pathway that would lead him to health and wellness. Instead of taking the high blood pressure drug, he went off the inhaler. Meanwhile, Bob's wife was growing increasingly concerned about his severe asthma attacks and insisted that he find a new doctor.

Bob found his way to my office serendipitously. When the shortwave band on his radio broke, he was unable to listen to his favorite radio station, so he turned on the AM band and found my radio show, *Health and Wellness Solutions*. Coincidentally, that morning I was talking about health problems that were similar to Bob's. He called my office and asked for the earliest available appointment.

When I first saw Bob, I didn't have to ask him how he felt. It was clear that he was in a health crisis. In fact, he was experiencing an early asthma attack, so I immediately gave him sublingual allergy-neutralizing drops. Here's how Bob describes the experience: "After three seconds I felt so good I couldn't believe it. I jumped off the table and held my arms out. For the first time in I don't know how long, maybe years, I held my arms straight out from right to left and went straight down on my knees and squatted, then I came back up, and didn't fall over. It took away the dizziness, the headache. I was just in shock."

Bob went through a series of skin tests to pinpoint his allergic sensitivities. Not surprisingly, he was highly allergic. I prescribed allergy drops to help neutralize Bob's allergies and prescribed a diet to help reduce his food allergies. He was also treated with natural thyroid and testosterone supplementation, therapies that will be discussed in later chapters.

Bob's transformation was truly remarkable. Before he began treatment, Bob strained to do one bench press at 135 pounds. Nine months later, he was able to do three sets of eight at this weight. From being barely able to walk on a treadmill for twenty minutes, he was now able to run for forty-five minutes. These are things he had never dreamed of being able to do.

On a recent visit Bob described how he was doing. "Dr. Hotze," he said, "did you realize that my first appointment with you was ten years to the day when my heart stopped? That appointment was the first day of my new life." He then gave me a compliment that would make my mother proud: "I thank God you think outside of the box."

CHAPTER 5

Yeast: The Fungus Among Us

When I first began practicing allergy medicine in 1989, I quickly learned that unmanaged allergies could cause a downward spiral of worsening health. The inflammation that occurs with allergies causes sinus congestion, which promotes bacterial growth, leading to recurrent sinus infections, for which the usual treatment is antibiotics. While these powerful drugs do kill harmful bacteria, they also kill good bacteria that serve useful functions in our bodies. This often results in a new problem: an overgrowth of the yeast *Candida albicans*.

Yeast overgrowth, a condition called candidiasis, can affect virtually any organ in the body, causing symptoms as varied as abdominal pain and headaches, fatigue and skin rashes, immune suppression and chemical sensitivity, and depression and joint pain. It's no wonder patients with unmanaged allergies eventually come to feel "sick all over." Nine times out of ten, I find that frequent antibiotic use and the resulting overgrowth of yeast is a major factor in their declining health.

FACTS ABOUT ANTIBIOTICS

- Doctors write about 100 million antibiotic prescriptions a year.
- Two of the top ten drugs prescribed in 2003 were antibiotics.
- A report by the National Institute of Medicine found that up to 50 percent of antibiotics are prescribed needlessly.
- Even if you've never taken antibiotics, you're likely to have ingested traces of them in dairy products and meat.
- Women are eight times more likely than men to be affected by yeast overgrowth. Higher antibiotic use (for bladder infections and treatment of acne) and the use of synthetic estrogen and birth control pills increase the risk for women.

ANTIBIOTICS ARE NO MAGIC BULLET

Though antibiotics are powerless against allergies and the viruses that cause colds, they are usually effective in treating acute bacterial sinus and bronchial infections. However, it isn't always easy to tell whether a patient is suffering from an allergic episode, a cold, or a sinus infection. As a result, physicians often prescribe antibiotics "just in case."

In addition, many physicians do not always differentiate between acute and chronic sinus infections before writing a prescription for an antibiotic. Yet a recent Mayo Clinic study found that most chronic sinus infections are not caused by bacteria, but by an immune system response to a fungus. Because antibiotics are effective only against bacteria, prescribing these drugs for a chronic fungal sinus infection is not appropriate.

Despite warnings about the development of antibiotic-resistant bacteria, physicians aren't prescribing fewer antibiotics. In fact, in one recent seven-year period, the number of antibiotic prescriptions written for sinus infections more than doubled. While antibiotic overuse is a serious public health issue, it is also an extremely important personal health issue. My office is filled with the records of patients who have been made ill by overuse of these drugs.

Physicians Ignore the Obvious

Jenny's story is typical. This thirty-one-year-old woman came to my office on her mother's advice after suffering years of progressively worsening health. Jenny had severe allergies and recurrent respiratory infections and had been on antibiotics for two years straight. A year before she consulted me she had undergone surgery for endometriosis. Jenny's gynecologist told her afterwards that she had the worst case of yeast overgrowth in her abdominal cavity that he had ever seen. Jenny was shocked when she saw the photos.

Jenny's gynecologist did not tell her that the antibiotics she had been taking were the cause of her yeast problem, nor did

Jenny's dermatologist, who prescribed antibiotics for her acne. By the time I saw Jenny, her yeast antibodies, measured by a blood test, were three times higher than normal. The symptoms she described were classic indicators of chronic candidiasis: abdominal pain and bloating, recurrent vaginal yeast infections, extreme fatigue, depression, and "brain fog." She told me that she was so exhausted she felt twice her age.

It was clear when I examined Jenny and reviewed her medical history that there were other factors contributing to her poor health. However, her severe yeast overgrowth was an immediate concern. Like the weeds that can destroy a flourishing garden, Jenny's overgrowth of yeast was depleting her energy, weakening her resistance to disease, and causing both physical and mental suffering. Restoring the normal balance of bacteria in her digestive tract was our number one priority.

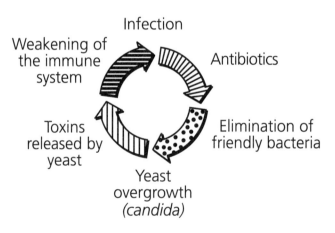

Antibiotics destroy good bacteria along with the bad, allowing yeast to proliferate in the digestive tract and vagina. Toxins released by yeast enter the bloodstream and impair immunity. Weakened immunity contributes to recurrent infections, leading to frequent antibiotic use, perpetuating the cycle.

Figure 2. The cycle of illness.

ANTIBIOTIC SHOTGUNS

As newborns, our large intestines are colonized by beneficial bacteria with tongue-twisting names like *Lactobacillus acidophilus* and *Bifidobacteria bifidum*. These bacteria, acquired from our mothers as we pass through the birth canal, perform a number of useful functions in our bodies. They manufacture B vitamins, aid in the digestion and absorption of food, and serve as sentries to help keep harmful bacteria at bay. Besides coexisting peacefully in the colon, beneficial bacteria also reside in the mucous membranes of the throat and in the vagina.

Antibiotics are more like shotguns than rifles, causing widespread damage rather than a clean hit. When you take a course of antibiotics, populations of all bacteria plummet—not just the harmful ones that are the target of the drug, but also the beneficial ones that keep you healthy. At the same time, yeast populations increase because they are not harmed by antibiotics that kill their normal bacterial competitors.

The effects of yeast overgrowth are wide-ranging. In the digestive tract, yeast can cause symptoms of cramping, bloating, constipation, and diarrhea. Women who take repeated courses of antibiotics often develop vaginal yeast infections as healthy bacteria are destroyed and candida proliferates. As yeast toxins are absorbed in the colon and enter the bloodstream, they cause symptoms beyond these sites. Fatigue, depression, inability to concentrate, headaches, muscle aches, joint pain, hives, skin rashes, athlete's foot—the list of yeast-related symptoms goes on and on.

Even worse, yeast produces toxins that depress your immune system, making you more reactive to allergies and more susceptible to infections. This often leads to more frequent use of antibiotics, the killing of more good bacteria, and more yeast overgrowth. This vicious cycle is hard to break. Sadly, it is a problem of which many mainstream physicians are completely unaware. Instead of addressing the underlying cause of their patients' poor health, they treat the individual symptoms, usually with the familiar "anti" drugs: antibiotics, antihistamines, antidepressants, anti-inflammatories, antispasmodics, and so forth.

Diagnosing Candidiasis

In my office, all new patients are given a blood test to measure levels of candida antibodies. While high levels of antibodies are indicative of yeast overgrowth, some patients with a severely depressed immune system do not respond appropriately to candida and instead show normal or even low levels of antibodies. For this reason, and because laboratory tests provide only a snapshot of a patient's health status, I rely much more on the patient's history and symptoms to determine the likelihood and extent of a yeast problem. (See appendix A for a questionnaire that can help you determine if you have yeast overgrowth.)

Each patient is asked questions relating to their history of infections and other illnesses, their diet, the symptoms they are experiencing, and their past and current use of antibiotics and other prescription drugs. For example, although antibiotics are the worst culprit in yeast syndrome, I also ask patients about their use of steroids and, in females, their use of birth control pills and estrogen. These drugs are known to stimulate yeast growth.

A history of recurrent infections is common in patients with candidiasis. The toxins produced by yeast impair immunity, as do the antibiotics prescribed to treat bacterial infections. A worsening of allergy symptoms, or the development of an allergy to yeast, can also occur in response to yeast overgrowth. Patients who used to tolerate alcohol might begin experiencing abnormal reactions such as flushing, headaches, sinus congestion, or itching skin. Sensitivity to tobacco smoke, perfumes, and other airborne chemicals may also develop.

Patients with yeast syndrome often crave sugar, bread, and other starchy foods. The reason? Yeast grows on sugar and on any food that can quickly be broken down into sugar. Cravings for sugar are both the cause and consequence of yeast overgrowth and are a primary target of treatment.

Yeast syndrome is a condition with multiple causes and multiple effects. For this reason, no single intervention will be effective in getting yeast under control, restoring the normal balance of healthy bacteria in the body, and restoring health. I have found that the most effective way of treating candidiasis is a three-pronged approach: eradicate, eliminate, and repopulate. Although I will talk about these steps as if they occurred in sequence, in reality you must undertake all three simultaneously in order to overcome this systemic illness and regain your health.

Step One: Eradicate

No garden can flourish if it has been overrun with weeds. Likewise, your body cannot function normally if it has been overtaken by yeast. Eradicating yeast is a crucial step in restoring health not only to your digestive tract but also to your entire body.

While there are over-the-counter agents such as garlic and caprylic acid that are helpful for eliminating yeast, my experience in treating thousands of patients with candidiasis has led me to believe that a more aggressive approach is necessary. In my office, most patients with candidiasis are prescribed an antifungal drug called nystatin. This drug has been in use for over fifty years and is a safe, effective agent for eradicating yeast in the colon. It is not absorbed systemically, and it does not affect the beneficial bacteria that normally inhabit the colon.

Patients stay on nystatin for one to three months or longer, depending on their symptoms and yeast antibody levels. Because nystatin only kills yeast in the spore form and its effects are confined primarily to the colon, we also prescribe a one- to two-week course of a systemic antifungal medication called Diflucan (fluconazole). This helps ensure that yeast cells in the mycelial stage are eradicated from the mucous membranes throughout the body.

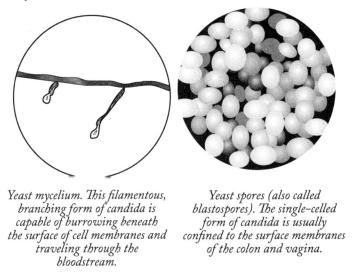

Yeast mycelium. This filamentous, branching form of candida is capable of burrowing beneath the surface of cell membranes and traveling through the bloodstream.

Yeast spores (also called blastospores). The single-celled form of candida is usually confined to the surface membranes of the colon and vagina.

Figure 3. Forms of *Candida albicans*.

Vaginal yeast infections are a common consequence of antibiotic overuse and candidiasis. Rather than using over-the-counter treatments that contain irritating chemicals, our patients are instructed to make a douche using three capsules of nystatin and three capsules of a *Lactobacillus acidophilus* supplement in warm water. Douching twice daily for two to three days usually eradicates the infection.

Onychomycosis, a fungal infection affecting the nails, is another common consequence of candidiasis. Because the most common prescription drugs for this condition, which are taken orally, are very hard on the liver, I rarely recommend them. A far safer treatment is topical tea tree oil *(Melaleuca alternifolia)*, which is effective not only for nail infections but also for fungal skin infections such as jock itch and athlete's foot. A 1994 study published in the *Journal of Family Practice* found that topical tea tree oil was as effective as the oral prescription drug Lotrimin (clotrimazole) in clearing up nail fungus. I recommend an even more effective topical preparation, which combines tea tree oil with liquid Diflucan (fluconazole) and DMSO. This combination solution, which is applied topically to the toenails daily, penetrates the nails and kills the fungus. It takes several months of use to eradicate nail fungus. The longer it has been present, the harder it is to treat effectively.

Step Two: Eliminate

Eradicating the yeast that is already present is only one element of a successful candida treatment program. You must also prevent yeast from regaining a foothold in your body.

Otherwise, while you may win the battle, you ultimately will lose the war.

To grow, yeast requires a specific environment—a moist, dark place with a constant food supply. This is a perfect description of your gastrointestinal tract. Fortunately, discouraging the growth of yeast doesn't mean that you have to go on a thirty-day fast. It does mean that you have to radically change your diet for at least this length of time in order to prevent yeast from growing.

The yeast-free, grain-free diet that I recommend eliminates dietary sources of yeast and other fungi, vinegar and fermented products, and sugar and carbohydrate-rich foods that provide nourishment to yeast. Here are the basics.

YEAST-FREE EATING PROGRAM

These foods are permitted throughout the one-month yeast-free eating program:
- Meats (chicken, beef, turkey, pork, lamb, venison, seafood)
- Vegetables (limit starchy vegetables such as squash, corn, carrots, etc.)
- Dried beans (black, red, kidney)
- Eggs (boiled, poached, scrambled, or fried with olive oil)
- Oatmeal (slow cooking; in recipes only)
- Lemons and limes
- Avocados
- Black olives
- Cold-pressed extra-virgin olive oil
- Nuts and nut butters
- Herbal teas
- Regular coffee and tea

For one month, avoid the following:
- Sugar and artificial sweeteners (aspartame, saccharin)
- Fruit juices, grapes, and bananas
- Breads, cereals, and baked goods
- Grains (corn, wheat, rye, millet, rice, barley)
- Potatoes
- Milk and milk products (cheese, yogurt, sour cream, ice cream)
- Soft drinks and decaffeinated beverages
- Wine, beer, and spirits
- Vinegar and products containing vinegar (pickles, green olives, salad dressings, soy sauce, mustard, mayonnaise, ketchup, etc.)
- Mushrooms
- Vegetable shortening, margarine, and partially hydrogenated oils

After two weeks, you may add:
- Fruits (except fruit juices, grapes, and bananas)
- Butter

Eliminating sugar can be the most difficult part of this diet, in part because so many foods contain added sugar. In addition to cane sugar and beet sugar, you will have to steer clear of honey, corn syrup, maple syrup, molasses, fruit sugar (fructose), milk sugar (lactose), and malt sugar (maltose), because yeast grows on sugar. Refined grains and starchy foods such as bread, pizza, pasta, cereal, potatoes, and rice are also off limits, because they can be quickly broken down into simple sugars.

Once you have successfully killed off the yeast through the use of antifungal medication and the yeast-free, grain-free diet, you can bring some of the foods back into your diet on a rotational basis. (See appendix D.)

Step Three: Repopulate

As I've mentioned several times in this chapter, the reason yeast gains the upper hand in patients who have taken antibiotics is that these drugs destroy healthy bacteria along with the harmful ones. Step three of this comprehensive anti-yeast program is to repopulate the colon with the beneficial bacteria that normally reside there.

This is easily accomplished by taking supplements of probiotics, including *Lactobacillus acidophilus, Bifidobacteria bifidum,* and other friendly bacteria. This is a must for patients with candidiasis, but whether you suffer from yeast overgrowth or not, taking a course of probiotics is also good preventive medicine whenever you're required to take an antibiotic for a bacterial infection.

A Word About "Yeast Die-Off"

Paradoxically, some patients begin to feel worse, not better, when they begin the anti-yeast program. Though this can be a disturbing experience, it is actually a sign that the treatment is working. These symptoms are the predictable result of yeast die-off, also called the Herxheimer reaction.

When large numbers of yeast cells die in a short period of time, the body has a difficult time detoxifying them quickly. As a result, yeast toxins enter circulation and can cause symptoms in the mucous membranes that cover the surfaces of most organs in the body, including the mouth, esophagus, stomach, intestines, sexual and urinary organs, sinuses, ears, and bronchi.

Each person's die-off reaction is different. In some patients, preexisting symptoms are exacerbated; in others, new symptoms appear. Symptoms can last anywhere from several days to two weeks. In some cases, reducing the dosage of nystatin is appropriate to slow down the die-off process and lessen the symptoms. Following the yeast-free, grain-free diet is critical to helping you weather this period.

Another measure that has proven helpful in our clinic is supplementing with sodium bicarbonate (baking soda) and potassium bicarbonate, which help neutralize the effects of toxins that are released by dying yeast cells. Try an 8-ounce glass of water with a tablespoon of baking soda. Over-the-counter Alka-Seltzer Gold is another option.

A diet high in simple carbohydrates, like bread products, and high in sugar can become addictive. When these are eliminated from the diet, withdrawal symptoms, similar to the symptoms of yeast die-off often occur. Be patient. This too will pass.

JENNY GOT HER LIFE BACK

If you have been suffering with chronic yeast overgrowth, this comprehensive anti-yeast program can yield rapid and sometimes surprising improvement in your physical and psychological well-being. Jenny, whose yeast overgrowth was the worst her gynecologist had ever seen, can attest to this. In six weeks on the yeast-free, grain-free diet, she lost ten pounds. As the populations of yeast in her body declined, her depression lifted, her ability to concentrate improved measurably, and her cravings for bread and sweets subsided. She began sleeping normally and awakened refreshed and eager to start the day.

In a recent follow-up interview, Jenny expressed excitement about the tremendous health gains she had achieved in just six short weeks. "My life was being taken away from me because of my poor health. To think that my life has been given back to me that quickly is just amazing. I'll be entering the seminary this fall, and I'm excited about the coming two years because I actually have an attention span, and I can concentrate on doing what I'm supposed to do."

Although I credit the anti-yeast program for much of Jenny's improvement, there was another aspect of her treatment that was likely a major factor in her resurgence of energy and well-being: natural thyroid replacement, using Armour Thyroid, to correct her hypothyroidism (low thyroid function). In the next chapter you will learn how this underdiagnosed, extremely common condition is robbing millions of women of their vitality.

CHAPTER 6

Hypothyroidism: The Hidden Epidemic

Before I entered the field of allergy medicine, I believed that hypothyroidism was a relatively rare condition in the United States. The introduction of iodized salt in the 1920s had virtually eliminated iodine deficiency, a major cause of hypothyroidism. In my sixteen-year career as a physician, I had seen only one case of myxedema, end-stage hypothyroidism, and that was during my internship at St. Joseph's Hospital in Houston in 1976.

Myxedema takes years to develop and most patients with hypothyroidism are identified and treated long before this late stage occurs. The patient I saw during my internship had inexplicably gone without medical care until his condition was so severe that he required hospitalization. My mentor, Dr. Fred, was able to diagnose this patient simply by looking at him lying in his hospital bed.

One night while I was on duty, I was called by this patient's wife to his room because he had quit breathing. I had to insert a breathing tube into his windpipe and attach the tube to a ventilator. He was then transferred to the intensive care unit where the chief resident, Dr. Charles Butler, gave him intravenous thyroid hormone. Despite this frightening episode and the severity of this patient's condition, he made a remarkable recovery. In fact, five days after his near-death experience, he was chasing a nurse around his hospital room.

Although this patient's dramatic improvement made a lasting impression on me, it wasn't until I entered the field of allergy medicine that the evaluation and treatment of hypothyroidism became a cornerstone of my medical practice. For that, I have to thank Richard Mabray, M.D., a physician from Victoria, Texas.

At the 1992 Pan American Allergy Society conference in Houston, I had the opportunity to visit Dr. Mabray, a very successful obstetrician and gynecologist who also treated allergies. Dr. Mabray advised me to read *Hypothyroidism: The Unsuspected Illness*, by Broda Barnes, M.D. I did, and the insights that I gained from Dr. Barnes's book changed not only my life but also the lives of thousands of patients that I have treated for hypothyroidism.

THE UNSUSPECTED ILLNESS

Broda Barnes was a brilliant physician who studied physiology at the University of Chicago in the 1930s. His doctoral dissertation concerned the role of the thyroid gland in rabbits. Dr. Barnes noted that when rabbits had their thyroid glands removed, their development was impaired. They soon became extremely lethargic, experienced hair loss, and contracted recurrent infections. If a rabbit was given supplemental thyroid hormone, its health improved dramatically. Without it, however, its lifespan was half the length of rabbits with intact thyroid glands.

After he received his Ph.D., Dr. Barnes went on to earn a medical degree from the University of Chicago Medical School. As a physician, Dr. Barnes encountered numerous patients who had been categorized by other physicians as hypochondriacs. After listening to his patients' multiple, vague complaints and examining them, it dawned on Dr. Barnes that these patients reminded him of the rabbits lacking thyroid glands that he had studied. He decided to supplement these patients with thyroid hormone. To his delight, most of the patients responded beautifully to this therapy. Their physical symptoms disappeared, and their energy and well-being significantly improved.

Dr. Barnes's book, based on nearly forty years of medical experience, was published in 1976—the same year that I had encountered the patient with myxedema. At that time, the medical profession viewed hypothyroidism as a relatively rare condition that was best diagnosed by measuring blood levels of thyroid hormones and best treated with synthetic hormones. Dr. Barnes's message was threefold: hypothyroidism was a common but too often unrecognized problem; blood tests were not very useful for diagnosing this condition; and natural desiccated thyroid hormone, such as Armour Thyroid, was the best form of treatment.

Since the release of his book, hypothyroidism has become a regular topic in women's magazines. However, despite the greater media attention that hypothyroidism now receives, most American women who have hypothyroidism remain undiagnosed. Even those who suspect that low thyroid function is the underlying cause of their fatigue, weight gain, depressed mood, brain fog, and other symptoms seldom get help from their physicians. The reason for this is that most physicians have been influenced by a herd mentality. They don't treat patients, they treat lab values.

But Dr. Barnes was right—lab tests aren't the best way to diagnose hypothyroidism or to assess whether treatment is working, as the following two stories demonstrate.

Brenda's Story

Brenda is a forty-year-old mother of two and a substitute teacher. Around the age of thirty-five, Brenda's health took a turn for the worse. She became depressed and was chronically exhausted, even though she exercised. She felt cold all the time, had recurrent infections, and began losing her hair. She was constipated despite the fact that she ate a high-fiber diet and drank plenty of water. And her libido had plummeted, a fact that distressed both her and her husband.

Within the course of a year, Brenda sought the care of a gynecologist, an internist, a gastroenterologist, and a family practitioner, trying to get help for her many problems. While some said she had symptoms of hypothyroidism, they all insisted that her blood tests were normal. Their diagnosis could be summed up in five words: "Nothing is wrong with you."

Brenda knew that something was physically wrong. As she told me later, "Two doctors told me that my fatigue and other problems were all age related. That was when I was thirty-five. I remember thinking, 'Thirty-five, give me a break. Maybe sixty-five!' I was always tired, even though I got a full night's sleep. I knew that I had some sort of a physical problem, if only I could find a doctor to figure it out."

Kathryn's Story

Kathryn's story parallels that of Brenda in many ways. This forty-four-year-old mother of three works as an executive administrator for a large corporation in Houston. Kathryn was diagnosed with hypothyroidism at the age of thirty-five and was prescribed a synthetic thyroid medication, Synthroid. Kathryn had taken Synthroid (levothyroxine sodium) daily for the past nine years, yet she still had numerous symptoms of a low thyroid condition.

Kathryn suffered from extreme fatigue and had problems with her thinking and short-term memory, which made it difficult for her to function in her career. When I asked her how she managed, she said, "I use every ounce of energy to make it through the week so I can rest up on the weekends, only to have to start all over again on Monday. My friends and family tell me that I am grumpy, but if they felt the way I do, I'm sure they would be grumpy too."

Kathryn told me that she had gained seventy pounds in the past decade, although she watched what she ate. "I've seen all kinds of doctors to try to figure out why I can't lose weight," she said. "I've been to a family practitioner, ob-gyn, endocrinologist, and even a nutritionist. The doctors gave me prescriptions for diet pills and told me to stay away from fatty foods. But I didn't eat those things anyway!"

Kathryn was extremely discouraged about her lack of energy and her inability to lose weight. She was also discouraged by the dismissive attitude of the physicians she had consulted. "It's all in your head," one doctor had told her. Another had said, "You're in your forties and it's time for your body to start changing. The way you feel is normal."

Kathryn told me that she knew her problem was hormonal, but her endocrinologist insisted that she was on the right dose of Synthroid because her blood tests were normal.

"But I don't feel normal," she told me.

THE SPARK PLUG INSIDE THE CELL

Both Brenda and Kathryn had significant health problems that were affecting their work performance, their personal lives, and their sense of well-being. Both had their problems dismissed by unsympathetic physicians who looked more closely at their blood tests than they did at the living, breathing human beings standing before them. After I had taken the time to listen to these women's stories, to question them about their symptoms and examine them, it was apparent to me that their problems were not in their head but in their cells, which were starved of energy.

Though you may think of the food you eat as a source of your energy, your body requires more than food to build and maintain itself. The energy currency inside your body is a molecule called adenosine triphosphate (ATP). Your cells generate ATP from glucose through a complex series of chemical reactions that require the presence of thyroid hormones.

Allow me to use an analogy to help you better understand how this process works. When you put gasoline in your car's tank, this simple act is not sufficient to make your car run. The gasoline must flow through the fuel line and into the engine's combustion chamber. Inside the combustion chamber, the spark plugs must give off a spark to rupture the bonds between the gasoline molecules, which releases energy. This energy then drives the pistons, making the car run. The excess energy is expelled through the tailpipe as heat.

In your body, thyroid hormone functions as the spark plug of the cell. It causes the combustion of glucose, converting the energy stored within its bonds into ATP, which fuels the cellular reactions that keep your body humming along. As in your car, the excess energy is generated as heat, which keeps your body warm.

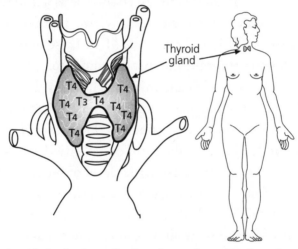

The thyroid gland, a butterfly-shaped organ located in the neck, produces two forms of thyroid hormone, T3 and T4. About 93 percent of its hormone production consists of T4; the remainder is T3.

Figure 4. The thyroid gland.

If you have an eight-cylinder car, but only seven spark plugs are working, then your car will run, but it will run rough and will not perform optimally. In the same way, if your cells do not have adequate levels of thyroid hormone, then the energy contained in the glucose molecule will not be efficiently converted to the energy molecule of the cell, ATP. The result will be a decrease in energy and lowered metabolism. If your thyroid gland were removed, your body would wind down like a toy soldier and cease to function altogether. Without thyroid replacement therapy, you would be dead within a year or two.

Other than surgical removal of the thyroid gland, there are two primary causes for a decline in the cells' supply of thyroid hormones: inadequate *production* of thyroid hormones by the thyroid gland and inadequate *absorption* of thyroid hormones by the cells. We're going to look at these two problems in greater detail in a moment. But before we begin, let me clarify one thing.

I have been speaking of thyroid hormone as if it were a single hormone. However, there are actually two thyroid hormones: triiodothyronine (T3) and thyroxine (T4). These hormones look quite similar except for the number of iodine atoms they contain: triiodothyronine has three and thyroxine has four, thus the names T3 and T4. The thyroid gland produces very different quantities of these two hormones. Approximately 93 percent of its thyroid hormone production is in the form of T4, and the remainder is in the form of T3. Despite its higher level of production within the thyroid gland, T4 is considered an inactive form of thyroid hormone. Only T3, or T4 that has been converted into T3 inside the cells, can be used to produce energy in our cells.

HO———⟨ ⟩——— O ——— ⟨ ⟩——— CO₂H

Triiodothyronine (T3)

Thyroxine (T4)

T3 (triiodothyronine) and T4 (thyroxine) have almost identical chemical structures. The only difference is that T3 contains three iodine (I) atoms and T4 contains four.

Figure 5. T3 and T4.

A Faulty Thermostat

Think of the thyroid gland as a heater. Just as your heater does not produce heat independent of the thermostat setting, your thyroid gland does not produce T3 and T4 independent of the signals from your internal thermostat, your pituitary gland. This tiny organ, located in the brain, is highly sensitive to changes in blood levels of thyroid hormone. When blood levels drop below a certain concentration, the pituitary gland responds by secreting thyroid-stimulating hormone (TSH). TSH travels to the thyroid gland, where it stimulates the production of more thyroid hormones.

The thyroid gland itself has no way of detecting when more thyroid hormone is needed. So if the pituitary gland is diseased and fails to produce TSH, the thyroid gland will not produce thyroid hormones, even when blood levels drop precipitously. Blood tests of a person with hypothyroidism due to a pituitary problem will show low levels of both TSH and T4, indicating that the thyroid gland is behaving "normally" in response to the subnormal activity of the pituitary gland.

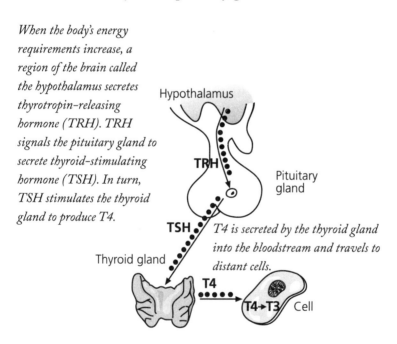

When the body's energy requirements increase, a region of the brain called the hypothalamus secretes thyrotropin-releasing hormone (TRH). TRH signals the pituitary gland to secrete thyroid-stimulating hormone (TSH). In turn, TSH stimulates the thyroid gland to produce T4.

Hypothalamus

TRH

Pituitary gland

TSH

Thyroid gland

T4 is secreted by the thyroid gland into the bloodstream and travels to distant cells.

T4

T4→T3   Cell

After it enters a cell, T4 must be converted into T3, the active form of thyroid hormone, in order to be used to fuel metabolic reactions.

Figure 6. From gland to cell.

I mentioned another cause of inadequate thyroid hormone production earlier: iodine deficiency. Remember, each thyroid hormone molecule contains three or four atoms of iodine. If your diet contains insufficient iodine, the thyroid gland will be unable to synthesize adequate amounts of thyroid hormone, even if the pituitary gland is sending an urgent message to do so. Iodine-deficiency hypothyroidism is characterized by an enlarged thyroid gland, or goiter. Blood tests will generally show high levels of TSH and low levels of T4, indicating that the pituitary gland is functioning normally but the thyroid gland is failing to respond to the signal. This type of hypothyroidism is now relatively rare in the US, although goiter regions still exist in many areas of the world.

Like Thieves in the Night

At the 1992 Pan American Allergy Society conference, Dr. Mabray advised me to evaluate my allergy patients for thyroid disease. "You will find that many of your allergy patients suffer from autoimmune thyroiditis," he said.

Autoimmune thyroiditis, also called Hashimoto's thyroiditis in honor of the scientist who first identified it, is similar to the allergic response in that it occurs when the immune system overreacts, launching an attack on something that normally would be considered innocuous. The difference is that, in autoimmune thyroiditis, the target is not an ingested or inhaled substance, but the body's own cells. Antibodies bind to the thyroid gland and prevent the manufacture of thyroid hormone. Antibodies also may bind to the circulating thyroid hormone, making it unavailable to the cells.

In 1992, I began testing all of my patients for thyroid antibodies and found that allergies and hypothyroidism traffic together like thieves in the night. A full 28 percent of my female allergy patients had this disease, as did 18 percent of my male allergy patients. This is much higher than the incidence found in the general population. In 1996, the American Academy of Otolaryngic Allergy awarded me the Sam Sanders Award for Clinical Research for my study of the relationship between autoimmune thyroiditis and allergic disorders.

A Uniquely Female Problem

Hypothyroidism affects women seven times more frequently than men. The higher incidence of genetically inherited autoimmune thyroiditis among women is one reason why. The effect of female hormonal imbalance is another.

The menstrual cycle is characterized by changing ratios of the female hormones estrogen and progesterone. During the first half of the cycle estrogen dominates, and during the second half progesterone dominates. However, as the ovaries age, women produce decreasing amounts of progesterone, resulting in a condition called estrogen dominance.

Estrogen dominance causes the liver to produce increasing levels of thyroid-binding globulin (TBG), a protein that has a strong attraction to circulating thyroid hormones. When TBG latches onto a thyroid hormone, the hormone is no longer free to enter into the cells and be used for metabolic reactions.

Even in the most ideal of circumstances, only 0.05 percent of thyroid hormone circulating in the bloodstream—a mere five parts in ten thousand—remains unbound and available to the cells. The remainder—a full 99.95 percent—is bound to TBG and other proteins in the blood. In women with estrogen dominance, the situation is even worse, due to the higher levels of TBG that are produced by the liver.

Birth control pills, pregnancy, and postmenopausal estrogen supplementation also increase levels of TBG, compounding the problem for women. In contrast, the male hormone testosterone has no effect on TBG and actually stimulates the conversion of the inactive thyroid hormone, T4, to the active thyroid hormone, T3, within the cells. It's no mystery why women are much more likely than men to experience low thyroid function.

DO YOU HAVE HYPOTHYROIDISM?

Because thyroid hormones promote the burning of glucose for energy, the most noticeable effects of hypothyroidism—fatigue, weight gain, and sensitivity to cold—have to do with a slowdown in energy and heat production. However, thyroid hormones also regulate tissue growth and development, help maintain blood pressure and fluid balance, and affect the workings of virtually every cell in your body. For this reason, a deficiency state can cause a wide range of symptoms.

The brain is highly sensitive to hormone depletion, and patients with low levels of thyroid hormones often experience depression and problems with concentration and short-term memory. Hair loss, dry skin, and brittle nails are common features of low thyroid function.

A deficiency of thyroid hormones can affect levels of sex hormones, causing menstrual abnormalities in women and a loss of libido in both sexes. Hypothyroidism can also impair fertility and, if it is present during pregnancy, can cause miscarriage, premature delivery, or stillbirth.

PHYSICAL SIGNS AND SYMPTOMS OF HYPOTHYROIDISM

- Fatigue
- Cold extremities
- Decreased sweating
- Muscle and joint pain
- Menstrual irregularities
- Miscarriages
- Recurrent infections
- Decreased mental sharpness, "brain fog"
- Hoarseness
- Dry skin
- Constipation
- Skin pallor, pastiness, and puffiness
- Brittle fingernails with ridging
- Low blood pressure
- Low basal body temperature
- Elevated cholesterol and extremities   triglycerides

- Weight gain
- Cold intolerance
- Headaches
- Enlarged thyroid gland
- Infertility
- Loss of libido
- Allergic disorders
- Depression or mood swings
- Slow speech
- Hair loss
- Fluid retention
- Enlarged tongue with teeth indentations
- Loss of hair on the outer edge of the eyebrows
- Slow pulse rate
- Tingling and/or numbness in

Depending upon the degree of hypothyroidism, a patient may have one, some, or all of these symptoms.

A constellation of symptoms such as these is highly suggestive of low thyroid function. Yet, as Brenda's and Kathryn's stories demonstrate, most physicians do not give these symptoms much credence. Instead, they rely on blood tests to diagnose hypothyroidism, and if the tests come out normal, the patient is labeled a hypochondriac or told that she is depressed and sent off with a prescription for an antidepressant.

If a physician relies solely on blood tests to determine whether or not a patient has hypothyroidism, then what is the purpose of the office visit? What do the clinical history of the patient and the findings from the physical examination really matter? Why not just draw the patient's blood for study and save her the time, expense, and humiliation of an office visit?

Dr. Fred had diagnosed a patient's myxedema simply by looking carefully at the patient lying in his hospital bed. He had encouraged me to consider every bit of information available to me, including the evidence of my own eyes and ears, when making a diagnosis. "Don't treat lab values," he had said. "Treat patients."

The single most important tool in determining a patient's thyroid status is a thorough review of the patient's symptoms and a physical examination. (See appendix A for the questionnaire we use to help determine if hypothyroidism is present.) Laboratory data can be helpful to confirm the diagnosis, but when the results of lab tests do not correspond to the patient's signs and symptoms, it is the lab tests that should be considered suspect—not the patient. Let me explain why.

PATIENTS DON'T LIE—LAB TESTS DO

I have a healthy skepticism of lab tests, based on my own clinical experience with these tests. The same blood samples from several of my patients have been sent to different labs for measurement of their thyroid hormone levels, and the results have varied by as much as 50 percent. The most that can be said about a lab test is that it is a snapshot of what is going on in the blood at one moment in time. However, thyroid hormone blood levels vary throughout the day and their actions are affected by disease processes, prescription drugs, other hormones that the body produces, and even environmental chemicals.

Also, the "normal laboratory range" of thyroid hormones is an arbitrary value, defined statistically as plus or minus two standard deviations from the mean. This so-called normal range is as wide as the Grand Canyon. In practice, it means that approximately 90–95 percent of the population will always fall within the normal range. However, I assure you that 90–95 percent of the population does not feel healthy, well, and full of energy.

Not only that, but the arbitrarily defined "normal" value has actually changed over time. Between 1991 and 2002, the normal laboratory range for the free thyroxine (free T4) blood test was lowered by 15 percent, from 0.90–2.00 ng/dl to 0.76–1.70 ng/dl. What this means is that an individual in 1991 who had a free T4 value of 0.80 ng/dl would have been classified by a conventional doctor as hypothyroid, but an individual with an identical T4 value in 2002 would be told that her thyroid function was in the normal range and would be denied treatment. Yet these two patients, separated in time by eleven years, likely would have had numerous symptoms in common—symptoms that are highly responsive to thyroid hormone replacement therapy.

DECLINING HORMONES = DECLINING HEALTH

Leaving aside the problems of conflicting lab test results and variable definitions of what is "normal," there is another reason why lab tests should not be the sole factor in determining whether an individual has hypothyroidism: thyroid hormone levels decline with age, with predictable effects on energy and well-being. It is the relative decline in your thyroid hormone level that matters, not your level compared to some arbitrarily defined standard.

Let's say that as a healthy twenty-five-year-old, your free T4 level was 1.60 ng/dl—the high end of the "normal" range. By the age of fifty, your free T4 level might be as low as 0.80 ng/dl—the low end of the "normal" range. This represents a 50 percent decline in the thyroid hormone that is available for use by your cells. Since thyroid hormones enable your cells to generate energy, is it any wonder that as your thyroid hormone level declines, your energy level also decreases?

If a doctor relied solely on a lab test to evaluate your thyroid function, he would tell you that your condition is "normal"—but you wouldn't feel normal with 50 percent less thyroid hormone. To ensure that you have plenty of energy and feel healthy, your doctor should strive to maintain your thyroid hormone level in the range that is optimal for you.

This is the approach I take with my patients. Yes, I do perform blood tests, primarily to measure free thyroxine (free T4) and to determine whether thyroid antibodies are present. I also look at the total cholesterol and LDL ("bad" cholesterol) levels because these are often elevated in patients with hypothyroidism. However, my primary criterion for diagnosis—and for evaluating the effects of treatment—is how the patient feels.

If you came to my office with symptoms indicative of hypothyroidism, even though your thyroid hormone levels might be in the so-called "normal" range, I would likely offer you a therapeutic trial of thyroid hormone replacement. I would start you on a very low dose and then slowly increase this until your symptoms diminish.

An individual with hypothyroidism must be treated gently, like a car on a cold winter's day. When you get into a cold car and start the engine, it often knocks. Cold air comes out of the heat vents. If you gun the accelerator, you might throw a rod in the engine. Instead, you let the engine warm up slowly and then take the car on the road. Likewise, in the use of thyroid supplementation, small doses are prescribed initially and increased gradually until the symptoms are relieved. The final dose varies from patient to patient.

HYPOTHYROIDISM AND HEART DISEASE

Dr. Broda Barnes was a brilliant scientist. When a friend of his experienced a heart attack in 1950, Dr. Barnes reviewed his medical history, searching for clues. He found that his friend had suffered from symptoms of hypothyroidism for years, but had not sought treatment. Could this have been a factor in his heart attack?

Dr. Barnes knew of the relationship between hypothyroidism and high cholesterol and realized that his patients who were being treated for hypothyroidism had a remarkably low rate of heart attacks, despite the fact that the incidence of heart attacks was rising in the general population.

This observation led him to conduct a twenty-year study of the relationship between supplemental thyroid hormone and reduced risk of heart attacks. He was fortunate to have a landmark study against which to compare the heart attack rate in his own patients: the Heart Disease Epidemiology Study, also known as the Framingham Study, which began in 1949 under the sponsorship of the National Heart Institute and which continues to this day. In this study, five thousand residents of Framingham, Massachusetts, were selected to be followed medically for the rest of their lives in order to determine the cause of heart disease. Each person was followed with annual medical examinations and blood work. Their diets, smoking habits, and lifestyles were documented. However, these patients did not receive supplemental thyroid hormone.

In 1970, Dr. Barnes had 1,569 patients on natural thyroid hormone who were observed for a total of 8,824 patient years. These patients were classified by age, sex, elevated cholesterol, and high blood pressure, and compared to similar patients in the Framingham Study. Based on the statistics derived in the Framingham Study, seventy-two of Dr. Barnes's patients should have died from heart attacks; however, only four patients had done so. This represents a decreased heart attack death rate of 95 percent in patients who received natural thyroid hormone—a truly remarkable finding.

Doctors often recommend that patients with an increased risk of heart attack take a daily aspirin supplement, pointing to studies suggesting that this will reduce the incidence of heart attacks by 28 percent. Why not consider using natural thyroid hormone supplementation to reduce the death rate from heart attacks? Remember thyroid production declines as we age. Fifty-year-olds produce one half the thyroid hormones that they made during their twenties.

WHICH FORM OF THYROID HORMONE
REPLACEMENT IS BEST?

Synthroid is the number one prescribed treatment for hypothyroidism. In 2002, it was the fourth most prescribed drug in the United States. But a drug's popularity is no guarantee of its efficacy, as Kathryn's experience with this synthetic hormone shows.

I had been trained to use synthetic thyroid drugs myself, but when I spoke with Dr. Mabray at the 1992 Pan American Allergy Society conference, I asked him which product he used. Dr. Mabray told me that he treated hypothyroidism with Armour Thyroid, a natural prescription thyroid supplement that he felt was much more effective than the synthetic thyroid drugs. While I had great respect for Dr. Mabray, I thought it wise to seek a second opinion. For that, I turned to Dor Brown, M.D., the patriarch and cofounder of the Pan American Allergy Society.

Dr. Brown lived in Fredericksburg, Texas, and even though he was in his eighties, at that time he had one of the largest allergy practices in the country. He is also one of the finest clinicians I have ever known. Although he is board certified in both ear, nose, and throat surgery and ophthalmology, his practice is multifaceted. Patients have traveled from all over the country seeking his expertise for a host of medical conditions.

When I asked Dr. Brown whether I should use Armour Thyroid or the synthetic thyroid replacement drugs, he recommended, "Use Armour Thyroid."

When I asked why, he retorted, "Because it works!"

My clinical experience in treating some six thousand patients over the past thirteen years has convinced me that Dr. Brown was absolutely right. Because thyroid and allergic disorders often go hand in hand, I have had the opportunity to evaluate many patients for allergic disorders who were already being treated for hypothyroidism with synthetic thyroid. Most of these patients had significant symptoms of low metabolic function, even while taking synthetic thyroid. Once these patients were converted to Armour Thyroid and given the appropriate dosage, their symptoms of hypothyroidism markedly improved.

There is a very good explanation for why so many people languish on synthetic thyroid. Synthroid, Levoxyl, Levothroid, and other levothyroxine sodium products contain only a synthetic version of T4, the inactive form of thyroid hormone. Taking T4 without T3 is like replacing only seven of the eight spark plugs in your car's engine. Your body's "engine" will run, but it will never function as well as it should.

In contrast, Armour Thyroid, which is obtained from the thyroid gland of pigs, contains the same thyroid hormone molecules that the body produces, T3 and T4, along with nutrients from the thyroid gland. Armour Thyroid is an FDA-approved product that is formulated according to the exacting standards of the United States Pharmacopoeia (USP). To ensure that the product is consistently potent from batch to batch and tablet to tablet, analytical tests are performed on the raw material and the actual tablets.

T3 + T4 = IMPROVED MOOD AND COGNITION

Given the choice, most patients with hypothyroidism would prefer to take a thyroid hormone product that includes both T3 and T4. This isn't just my observation: it's the conclusion of a landmark study published in the *New England Journal of Medicine* on February 11, 1999. In this ten-week study, patients with hypothyroidism were randomized into two groups. One group received isolated T4 preparations for the first five weeks and a combination of T3 and T4 for the last five weeks; in the second group, this sequence was reversed. All of the capsules looked alike, so the patients were unaware of which treatment they were receiving during each five-week period.

On the last day of each five-week period, patients were administered standardized psychological tests to assess their levels of depression, anxiety, anger, and other traits. They were also given cognitive tests of memory, attention, learning, and other functions. On eleven of seventeen measures of mood and cognition, there was no significant difference between the two treatments. However, on six measures, the combination of T3 and T4 proved superior to isolated T4. In particular, when patients received both thyroid hormones, their symptoms of fatigue, depression, and anger were significantly improved, and they performed better on tests of attention, mental flexibility, and learning.

In addition to performing better on standardized tests, patients rated their own mood and physical symptoms as significantly improved on the combination product in comparison to isolated T4. When asked which treatment they preferred, the majority preferred the combination product, stating that they had more energy, could concentrate more easily, and simply felt better.

Synthetic Thyroid Drugs: A Tarnished History

Effectiveness is the most important criterion in choosing a thyroid replacement product. But equally important is the safety of the product. Here again, natural thyroid has proven superior. Natural thyroid extracts have been in use for over a century and were approved by the FDA in 1939, a year after the passage of the Food, Drug, and Cosmetic Act. Synthroid, Levothroid, Levoxyl, and other synthetic T4 products entered the market years later without FDA approval, under the mistaken assumption that these products were not new drugs and that their manufacturers were not required to prove their safety or effectiveness.

However, in 1997, the FDA ruled that oral levothyroxine sodium products were indeed "new drugs" and that manufacturers who wanted to continue marketing these products must submit a new drug application for approval. This decision was based on a long history of potency and stability problems with these drugs. In fact, between the years 1991 and 1997, there were ten recalls of levothyroxine sodium tablets, involving more than 100 million tablets. These recalls occurred primarily because these products had a lower potency than claimed or had lost their potency before their expiration dates. In some cases, patients required hospitalization due to problems with their thyroid medication.

Despite this tarnished history, many physicians continue to prescribe Synthroid and other brands of synthetic thyroid hormone and remain opposed to Armour Thyroid. If synthetic thyroid hormone costs twice as much and is less effective, why do they use it? In my opinion, it is largely due to the massive marketing campaigns of the pharmaceutical companies that hold patents on these drugs. Because naturally occurring substances, including thyroid hormone, cannot be patented, these products have a lower profit margin, and the companies that make them do not have millions of dollars at their disposal for marketing. It is a battle of David versus Goliath. In this case, it is Goliath, the pharmaceutical industry, known as Big Pharma, that wins. The loser is the patient who is prescribed the less effective, more expensive product.

Two Happy Endings

Kathryn was one of the millions of patients who were mismanaged because of conventional medicine's bias against natural thyroid. Fortunately, when I switched her from Synthroid to Armour Thyroid, every aspect of her health improved dramatically. As she put it, "Mentally, I feel super. Physically . . . well, let me put it to you this way—I went from a size eighteen to a size eight." Kathryn was a fashion merchandising major in college, and she is thrilled to be able to go into a store and find clothes in her size. Her skin is no longer dry, her hair is thicker and fuller, and she feels more attractive and more confident. Even her friends have noticed the difference and have commented on how much happier she seems.

Brenda has also made a dramatic turnaround since beginning Armour Thyroid supplement therapy. "My energy has gone up from a two to a nine out of ten," she said. "Instead of directing my children's activities from the couch, I now get up with them in the morning and help them get ready for school." She also has more energy to do things during the day with friends. And now that her thyroid hormones are at an optimal level, Brenda no longer suffers from low libido—a change that both she and her husband appreciate.

When I asked Brenda if she had any advice for other women suffering from low energy and depression, she said, "It may take some detective work and some perseverance, but if you know that you have a health problem, keep searching until you find a doctor who will listen to you. Try different doctors until you find one who is willing to treat your underlying problem and not dismiss you as a hypochondriac. You'll know it was worth the trouble when you finally start to feel better."

CHAPTER 7

Natural Female Hormones: The Missing Link

After several years as an allergist, I began to notice an interesting pattern among my allergy patients. While my male patients typically had a lifelong history of allergies, many women were consulting me for help with allergies that had appeared, seemingly out of the blue, in midlife. For some women, childbirth seemed to be the trigger. For others, the onset of allergies was associated with a change in their menstrual cycles.

It became obvious to me that there must be a relationship between allergic disorders and female hormone fluctuations in midlife. However, I was an allergist, not a gynecologist. When I determined that a woman needed help with hormonal problems, I referred her to a gynecologist. But one day after work, I was sitting at my desk going through my mail when I came across a monograph by Julian Whitaker, M.D., on the therapeutic use of natural hormones. Because I was having great success treating hypothyroidism with natural thyroid replacement, I was eager to read what Dr. Whitaker had to say about this topic.

That evening at home, I read the chapter on natural thyroid. Dr. Whitaker's writings confirmed my own experience in treating patients with low thyroid function. Symptoms, not blood tests, are the best way to diagnose and manage hypothyroidism, he wrote, and natural thyroid extracts such as Armour Thyroid are the best way to treat this very common condition.

Dr. Whitaker's monograph contained chapters on other hormones, including estrogen, progesterone, testosterone, dehydroepiandrosterone (DHEA), and growth hormone. I read them all. By the end of the evening, I had a much greater appreciation of the therapeutic potential of hormones than I had just twenty-four hours earlier. I also had a much better understanding of the difference between natural hormones and the counterfeit hormones produced by drug companies.

A Patient Teaches Me

There is an old adage that states, "When the student is ready, the teacher will appear." And I was ready.

The day after I read Dr. Whitaker's monograph, I walked into Guest Room 2 at my center and there, sitting on the examination table, was Linda, a long-time patient of mine in her late thirties. She held out an audiocassette and said, "Dr. Hotze, would you like to learn about natural progesterone therapy? This is a tape by Dr. John Lee."

"That's interesting," I replied. "I just spent last night reading about natural progesterone and would be very interested in listening to what this doctor has to say about its use."

On my thirty-minute drive home that evening, I listened to the tape. Dr. Lee had been recommending natural progesterone supplementation to his female patients for almost twenty years with amazing results. On his audiotape, he explained how premenstrual complaints, reproductive difficulties, and menopausal symptoms could be triggered by the inevitable decline in a woman's production of progesterone, beginning in her midthirties.

Dr. Lee's descriptions of his patients' symptoms were the same problems about which my patients were complaining. "Natural progesterone could be the missing link that could help these women," I thought.

The next day, I reached Dr. Lee by phone in California and asked him, "Where in the world do I get natural progesterone?"

Dr. Lee replied that progesterone could be purchased with a prescription through a compounding pharmacy. A few days later, a local compounding pharmacist, Phil Pylant, dropped by my office to introduce himself and offer his services. It turned out that Phil was a highly respected compounding pharmacist who taught other pharmacists how to compound prescriptions. Phil told me that he was not only familiar with natural female hormones, but that he could also compound natural progesterone and the natural human estrogens (estradiol, estrone, and estriol) for my patients.

COMPOUNDING PHARMACY

The compounding of medications from bulk ingredients for individual patients, as deemed appropriate by a prescribing physician, is the historic practice of pharmacy and has been occurring since the inception of the profession of pharmacy, centuries ago. Drug compounding is the process by which a pharmacist prepares a medication, prescribed by a physician, to meet an individual patient's need. The practice of drug compounding is also known as compounding pharmacy.

The dosage or route of administration of compounded bioidentical hormones, such as natural progesterone, varies from that of commercially available drugs and is customized for each individual patient. On the other hand, drugs manufactured by pharmaceutical companies are mass produced and distributed to wholesalers who in turn sell to pharmacies for resale to the public. These drugs have limited dosage strengths and means of administration. They are not tailored for a specific patient. There is no direct personal interaction between the pharmaceutical manufacturer and the physician, pharmacist, or patient.

Pharmacies that compound bioidentical hormones purchase these hormones in bulk from pharmaceutical companies and laboratories that are registered and governed by the Food and Drug Administration (FDA).

Natural, bioidentical human hormones cannot be patented because they occur in nature. Drug companies make their profits by creating and patenting chemicals that never before existed in nature. This allows the drug companies to have a proprietary product that no one else can produce for at least seventeen years. Owning the patent rights to a drug enables the pharmaceutical company to advertise and sell that drug without competition, thus dramatically increasing profits.

In order for women to receive bioidentical hormones in the appropriate dosage, they must be prescribed for them by a physician experienced in their use. Few, if any, chain pharmacies specialize in compounding bioidentical hormones. There are many small, independent community pharmacies that dabble in compounding. However, for my patients, I always recommend that they obtain their compounded bioidentical hormones from pharmacies that specialize in compounding bioidentical hormones.

"THE BLACK CLOUD LIFTED"

The first woman for whom I prescribed natural female hormones was Louise. Louise, the wife of a minister, had originally consulted me for help with her chronic bronchitis, for which she had been taking antibiotics almost year-round. She also had terrible headaches, felt cold even in warm weather, and was concerned about her irregular heartbeat.

Allergy testing revealed that Louise was highly allergic to corn, which was causing her headaches. Based on her history and examination, I also determined that Louise suffered from functional hypothyroidism, which was the reason for her low body temperature and her slow and irregular heartbeat. Once Louise began taking Armour Thyroid, her heartbeat stabilized and she no longer felt cold all the time. And as long as she avoided corn, she no longer experienced debilitating headaches. However, she still suffered from irritable and depressed moods, which she described as a "black cloud" hanging over her head.

Louise underwent a total hysterectomy in her early thirties and had been on Premarin, horse estrogen unbalanced by progesterone, for nearly twenty years. Her depression and irritability began after her hysterectomy, but none of the doctors she consulted acknowledged that the removal of her reproductive organs and her use of Premarin could be blamed for her moodiness. They simply wrote her prescriptions for antidepressants. When the side effects of these drugs became unbearable, Louise stopped taking them.

When I saw Louise for a checkup shortly after reading Dr. Whitaker's monograph and listening to Dr. Lee's tape, it occurred to me that the counterfeit hormones that Louise had been taking for the past twenty years might be contributing to her emotional problems. Since Phil Pylant had already agreed to compound natural hormones for me, I advised Louise to stop taking Premarin, and I wrote her two prescriptions for the natural, bioidentical hormones progesterone and Bi-Est (bi-estrogen).

When Louise returned for follow-up two months later, she was beaming. She could hardly wait to tell me how much better she felt. "When I started using the progesterone, it felt like my body was receiving something it had been missing for twenty years," she said. "The black cloud that had been hanging over my head was lifted. I was so excited that I called my daughter, who had been experiencing the same troubles I had when I was her age. Her doctor had already suggested that she have a hysterectomy. I told her not to make the same mistake that I had made, but instead, to give natural progesterone a try."

She had even called her own mother, who had been a recluse in her house for the past ten years, and advised her to start on natural progesterone. "My sister called me two weeks ago," she reported, "and asked me what in the world I had given to our mother. I asked her why, and she told me that Mother was throwing a party for the neighbors. She said she couldn't remember Mother ever being so happy."

Why Estrogen Dominance Occurs

Louise, her daughter, her mother, and millions of other women of all ages and backgrounds share a common plight: they suffer from a condition known as estrogen dominance. To function optimally, the female body requires an optimal balance of estrogens (a trio of related hormones called estradiol, estrone, and estriol) and progesterone. Estrogen dominance occurs when the hormonal balance is shifted in favor of the estrogens. This condition just as correctly could be called progesterone deficiency.

How does this happen? For the most part, it is the inevitable result of the aging process. A woman's ovaries generally function best between a few years after puberty until around age thirty. However, as a woman ages, so do her ovaries. By the time a woman reaches thirty-five years of age she is over halfway through her menstrual life and her ovarian function begins to falter.

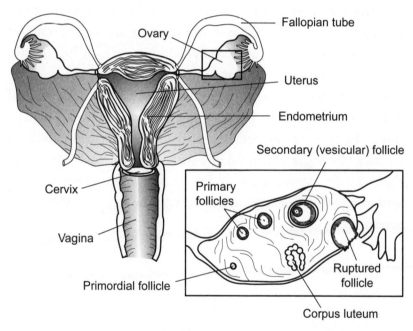

Each of the ovaries contains numerous follicles, which hold a woman's eggs. At ovulation, a mature (vesicular) follicle ruptures, releasing its egg. The follicle is then transformed into a progesterone-producing corpus luteum. If ovulation does not occur, no corpus luteum forms, and no progesterone is made.

Figure 7. The female reproductive organs.

The ovaries are the primary site for the production of both the estrogens and progesterone. But while both estrogen and progesterone levels decline with age, progesterone declines much more dramatically. By menopause, a woman's progesterone level is likely to be a mere $1/120$ of the level she experienced in her early twenties. In contrast, her postmenopausal estrogen level may remain at 40 percent of the level she experienced in early adulthood, because even when her ovaries no longer produce estrogen, her fat cells continue to do so. Thanks to this additional source of estrogen, an obese postmenopausal woman may have higher estrogen levels than a thin premenopausal woman.

Another reason why estrogen dominance becomes more common with age is that as a woman ages she begins to have anovulatory cycles, menstrual cycles during which her ovaries do not release eggs. When a woman does not ovulate, her ovaries produce no progesterone at all. The stimulatory effects of estrogen unopposed by progesterone can cause the endometrial lining to become abnormally thickened, resulting in heavier periods, clotting, and painful menstrual cramps. As women enter their thirties, anovulatory cycles become more common, and symptoms of estrogen dominance become progressively more severe.

Other Causes of Estrogen Dominance

While estrogen dominance is usually a progressive condition that develops as women move through their menstrual lives, it is virtually inevitable after a hysterectomy. As with natural menopause, surgically induced menopause obliterates progesterone production—immediately, rather than over years. Even if the ovaries have been spared the surgeon's knife, ovarian dysfunction or atrophy commonly occurs within two years following removal of the uterus, causing a predictable decline in progesterone levels.

Bilateral tubal ligation also can lead to a decline in the production of hormones by the ovaries. This procedure, in which the fallopian tubes are cut, burned, or tied off to prevent pregnancy, cuts off a portion of the blood supply to the ovaries. Many women who have undergone this procedure develop bilateral tubal ligation syndrome with symptoms of estrogen dominance.

Estrogen dominance can also occur following childbirth. During pregnancy, the placenta produces progesterone at levels that are many times higher than a woman's body normally produces. When the baby is delivered and the placenta is expelled, there is a precipitous drop in the progesterone level. However, estrogen levels remain high. Unless the ovaries can produce adequate amounts of progesterone to balance the estrogens, estrogen dominance is likely to occur.

Another factor contributing to estrogen dominance is the presence of xenoestrogens in our bodies. Xenoestrogens are found in petrochemical products such as plastics, herbicides, pesticides, soaps, clothing, industrial by-products, and countless other manufactured goods. The prefix "xeno" means alien, an apt description of these synthetic chemicals, which pollute the water, air, soil, and animal and plant life on this planet. Xenoestrogens can cause estrogenic effects even in doses on the level of a billionth of a gram, and because they are stored in the fat cells of our bodies, most of us carry a significant burden of these toxic chemicals.

Oral contraceptives are another common cause of estrogen dominance, because they work by suppressing ovulation and ovarian function. Keep in mind that a woman who is not ovulating produces no progesterone in her ovaries. Oral contraceptives contain progestins, not progesterone. Like xenoestrogens, synthetic progestins are alien to a woman's body, and although they target the same cell receptors that progesterone targets, their effects do not perfectly mimic those of the natural hormone. In fact, they depress the body's production of natural progesterone, leading to estrogen dominance and its associated symptoms.

THE NORMAL MENSTRUAL CYCLE

A normal menstrual cycle lasts twenty-eight days. The first day a woman starts her period is day one of her menstrual cycle. During the first fourteen days of the menstrual cycle the ovaries make increasing amounts of the estrogens. The function of these hormones is to stimulate the growth of the endometrial lining, the tissue that covers the inner surface of the uterus. This two-week period during which estrogen hormones are highest is termed the proliferative stage.

Midway through a woman's cycle, around day fourteen, one of her two ovaries will produce an egg. This is called ovulation. After ovulation, the ruptured follicle from which the egg has been released is transformed to a corpus luteum and begins producing progesterone as well as a small amount of testosterone. Both progesterone and testosterone, which peak just after ovulation, stimulate a woman's desire for sexual relations.

The portion of the menstrual cycle that follows ovulation, called the secretory phase, is orchestrated by progesterone. Progesterone's primary function is to mature the endometrial lining, preparing it for a potential pregnancy. Progesterone's importance to pregnancy is suggested by its name, which literally means "promoting gestation." If the egg fails to be fertilized and no pregnancy occurs, the production of both progesterone and the estrogen hormones dramatically falls at the end of the twenty-eight-day menstrual cycle. The endometrial lining is sloughed, leading to a period.

This cycle repeats itself over and over again during a woman's menstrual life, which extends from the time her periods begin at puberty until her periods cease at menopause.

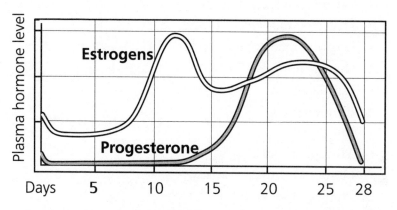

Levels of estrogen rise during the first half of the menstrual cycle, promoting the buildup of the endometrium, the inner lining of the uterus. After ovulation, progesterone levels rise, preparing the endometrium for implantation of an embryo. If pregnancy does not occur, levels of progesterone decline dramatically, triggering menstruation.

Figure 8. The normal menstrual cycle.

SYMPTOMS OF ESTROGEN DOMINANCE

Symptoms of estrogen dominance range from mildly annoying to severe. When a woman consults a physician for help with these symptoms, she is generally given two options: surgery, usually a hysterectomy, or prescription drugs, most often counterfeit hormones that actually worsen the problem. Rarely is she told that her problem is likely the result of estrogen dominance and that natural, bioidentical progesterone could alleviate her symptoms.

COMMON SYMPTOMS AND DISORDERS ASSOCIATED WITH ESTROGEN DOMINANCE

- Severe menstrual cramps
- Heavy periods with clotting
- Irregular menstrual cycles
- Uterine fibroids
- Ovarian cysts
- Endometriosis
- Infertility
- Multiple miscarriages
- Fibrocystic breast disease
- Premenstrual breast tenderness
- Premenstrual fluid retention and weight gain
- Anxiety, panic attacks, or depression
- Premenstrual mood swings
- Premenstrual headaches
- Migraines
- Decreased libido

While these symptoms may be common, they are not normal. They are indications of declining ovarian function and the resulting imbalance of estrogen and progesterone. If you suffer from any of these problems, you owe it to yourself to find a doctor who is experienced in treating female hormonal imbalances with natural, bioidentical hormones.

A Thirty-Year History of Suffering

Gail had always suffered from painful periods with heavy bleeding. At the age of eighteen, she was prescribed oral contraceptives to reduce her heavy menstrual flow. She remained on contraceptives until the age of thirty-two, when she became concerned about their link to cancer and discontinued them. At that time she began experiencing a heavy vaginal discharge, which seemed to coincide with her menstrual cycle. She also experienced a return of her painful cramps and heavy bleeding. And although she had lived in the same geographic region for years, she began to develop allergy symptoms.

Over the next ten years, Gail's allergies became more severe, so by the time she was forty-two, her symptoms persisted even when she took a prescription allergy drug. Her menstrual symptoms continued to worsen, and she began experiencing premenstrual breast tenderness and bloating. When her father died a year later, Gail's health went into a downward spiral. She contracted recurrent colds and suffered from mood swings and insomnia. She also began putting on weight.

Beginning in her thirties, Gail consulted a number of physicians for help with her premenstrual symptoms, painful periods, and other health problems. The responses of these physicians were at best unsympathetic and at worst insulting. One physician told her the heavy vaginal discharge was caused by her underwear. Another told Gail that she suffered from PMS— as if Gail didn't know that—and advised her to take vitamin B6, drink lots of fluids, and keep her chin up.

Gail underwent two highly sensitive Pap smears during this ten-year period, both of which came back with a diagnosis of "high estrogen effect." Yet neither of the physicians who had performed these tests told Gail that she was estrogen dominant and that natural, bioidentical progesterone could help alleviate her symptoms. A gynecologist that Gail consulted was pleased to tell her that the antidepressant Prozac could now be prescribed for PMS and urged her to make an appointment with a psychiatrist.

Gail had moved to the Houston area with her husband when she was forty-six. A female ob-gyn whom she consulted suspected that Gail's severe menstrual pain was caused by endometriosis and recommended that she undergo diagnostic laparoscopy. This procedure confirmed that Gail had endometriosis, which had spread to the bladder and had caused the colon to adhere to the uterus. She was once again put on oral contraceptives to reduce her menstrual flow.

One day, Gail happened to hear me speaking about female hormone problems on my radio program. She immediately called and made an appointment. When I sat down with her to discuss her symptoms, she told me that she was still experiencing menstrual cramps and premenstrual breast tenderness, along with some new symptoms, including low libido, intermittent hot flashes, premenstrual mood swings, and heart palpitations. In addition, she suffered from sinus headaches, cold hands and feet, restless sleep, decreased energy, and allergies to certain foods, pollens, and molds.

It was evident just from listening to Gail's description of her symptoms that she was estrogen dominant, even though she was also experiencing symptoms of menopause such as hot flashes. I suspected that she had functional hypothyroidism as well. After examining her and performing allergy testing, I prescribed natural, bioidentical estrogen and progesterone, Armour Thyroid, and sublingual allergy drops to address the underlying causes of her health problems.

A year and a half later, Gail was a vibrant woman. She was twenty-eight pounds lighter and radiated energy and well-being. Her sinus headaches had vanished, as had her hot flashes. She slept restfully and her moods were upbeat.

ESTROGEN DOMINANCE AND THE REPRODUCTIVE ORGANS

Gail's story reads like a textbook case of estrogen dominance. Her painful periods and heavy bleeding are classic symptoms of a relative excess of estrogen. As I mentioned earlier, estrogen is a stimulative hormone, and too much of this hormone causes overgrowth of endometrial tissue. Estrogen also makes the blood clot more easily. When large clots of blood are passed during menstruation, the result is severe cramping.

Endometriosis, which afflicted both Gail and Louise, is another condition in which estrogen dominance plays a major role. This painful condition occurs when cells that make up the inner lining of the uterus, the endometrium, form colonies outside of the uterus. These endometrial implants may attach to the uterus, fallopian tubes, colon, bladder, or other organs. Despite their position outside of the uterus, they respond to estrogen just as the cells within the uterine lining do. They multiply, swell with blood, and then bleed into the surrounding tissues during the menstrual period. Because the blood has nowhere to go, it can cause inflammation, scar tissue, and adhesions.

Estrogen also fuels the growth of uterine fibroids. These noncancerous growths shrink at menopause when estrogen levels decline. However, long before this occurs, a hysterectomy is usually recommended to women with symptomatic fibroids. In fact, fibroids are the number one reason for hysterectomies, even though in many cases it is possible to remove the fibroids and leave the uterus intact. Few women are given this option, and fewer still are given a therapeutic trial of natural, bioidentical progesterone to determine if this will alleviate their pelvic pain and other symptoms and enable them to avoid surgery altogether.

Like the uterus, the breasts are highly sensitive to the stimulatory effects of natural estrogen, counterfeit estrogens, and xenoestrogens. The premenstrual breast pain and tenderness that Gail began experiencing in her early forties is a classic symptom of estrogen dominance. Fibrocystic breast disease is another. This condition is characterized by lumps in the breasts that are noncancerous but very painful.

ESTROGEN DOMINANCE AND THE THYROID GLAND

As I mentioned in the previous chapter, hypothyroidism affects women seven times more frequently than men. The epidemic of estrogen dominance among women in this country is the cause of this disparity. When estrogen levels are high, the liver produces high levels of thyroid-binding globulin (TBG), a protein that binds to thyroid hormones in the blood and prevents them from being taken up by the cells. Birth control pills, pregnancy, and counterfeit estrogens prescribed during and after menopause also cause estrogen dominance and increased levels of TBG.

Women suffering from estrogen dominance may have a normally functioning thyroid gland that produces adequate amounts of thyroid hormone, and blood tests to measure levels of thyroid hormone and thyroid-stimulating hormone may be read as "normal." However, because the hormone is bound to and inactivated by circulating proteins, little of it is actually getting into the cells. A physician who relies solely on blood tests for diagnosis is likely to tell a woman that there is nothing wrong with her, despite the fact that her symptoms all point to a state of functional hypothyroidism.

I have said it before, but it bears repeating: Listening to the patient's symptoms rather than relying on blood tests is the best way to diagnose and treat hormonal problems. This is true not only of thyroid problems, but also of problems relating to the female hormones. Unlike body temperature, which varies little from day to day in a healthy person, hormone levels can vary widely, even within the same twenty-four-hour period. This is especially likely to occur among women in their premenopausal years.

ESTROGEN DOMINANCE AND THE BONES

Conventional thinking attributes osteoporosis to the decline in estrogen hormones that occurs in a woman's postmenopausal years. As it turns out, conventional thinking is wrong. Women begin losing bone mineral density years before menopause, and it is progesterone, not estrogen, that is crucial to preventing osteoporosis.

If estrogen were the most important hormone in maintaining bone health, then women would maintain their peak bone density until their fifties. They would experience bone loss only after menopause, when estrogen levels decline dramatically. However, this is not the case. A woman attains her peak bone density at approximately thirty years of age, after which she begins to lose bone at a rate of about 1–1.5 percent per year. While it is true that bone loss accelerates at menopause, this is a temporary phenomenon. Within three to five years, the rate of bone loss slows to premenopausal levels.

THE DANCE OF FEMALE HORMONES

Effects of Progesterone	Effects of Estrogen
• Matures the uterine lining and prevents excess tissue buildup	• Stimulates growth of the uterine lining
• Inhibits breast tissue overgrowth	• Causes growth of breast tissue
• Increases metabolism, promoting weight loss	• Promotes fat storage and weight gain
• Mobilizes fluid and decreases swelling	• Promotes fluid retention
• Thins the blood, preventing blood clots	• Causes thickening of the blood
• Stimulates the production of new bone	• Slows bone breakdown
• Enhances the action of thyroid hormones	• Reduces bioavailability of thyroid hormones
• Increases the sex drive	• Inhibits the sex drive

As this comparison demonstrates, the decline in progesterone levels that occurs beginning in a woman's midthirties is a much more critical factor in causing bone loss than the decline in estrogen levels that occurs at menopause. This is due to the interaction of progesterone and estrogen with specialized bone cells called osteoclasts and osteoblasts.

Osteoclasts are responsible for breaking down old bone, while osteoblasts build new bone. "Out with the old, in with the new" is your body's way of replacing worn-out bone cells with new, healthy cells. However, this only occurs when the activity of osteoclasts is balanced with that of osteoblasts.

Estrogen helps slow bone loss by curbing the activity of bone-dissolving osteoclasts, but it has no effect on osteoblasts. On the other hand, progesterone attaches to specialized receptor sites on the surface of the osteoblasts and stimulates bone-building activity.

The prevention of osteoporosis is yet another reason that I recommend women supplement with natural progesterone beginning in their midthirties.

Estrogen Dominance and the Brain

Louise, the first woman to whom I prescribed bioidentical hormones, suffered from depressed and irritable moods from the time of her hysterectomy at the age of thirty until she began using progesterone more than twenty years later.

Gail made it into her forties with her uterus intact before she began experiencing depression, mood swings, and emotional fragility. Both Louise and Gail attempted to pinpoint the source of their emotional problems in their stressful lives, but they also had the feeling that something was not right in their bodies, and that this something had to do with their hormones.

They were correct.

On the biochemical level, mood is largely the result of the balance of neurotransmitters—especially serotonin, dopamine, and norepinephrine—in the brain. Low levels of one or more of these chemical messengers are common in patients with depression. But levels of these and other neurotransmitters can be affected by hormonal variations. For example, the mood-elevating neurotransmitter norepinephrine is inactivated by an enzyme called monoamine oxidase (MAO), and when levels of MAO are high, the resulting decline in bioavailable norepinephrine can induce depression. This process can be reversed by estrogen, which inhibits MAO and frees up more norepinephrine.

On the other hand, chronically elevated levels of estrogen can actually induce depression and anxiety by causing functional hypothyroidism. When thyroid hormone cannot be adequately assimilated into the cells, cellular oxygen declines. This is bad news for the brain, which uses a full 25 percent of the oxygen you breathe. Hypothyroidism also results in a slowdown of cellular metabolism, which causes a drop in levels of the neurotransmitter gamma-aminobutric acid (GABA). GABA is a calming neurotransmitter, which prevents the brain from being overwhelmed by stimulation. Extremely low levels of GABA can cause epileptic seizures, but even moderately low levels are linked to mood swings, anxiety, and panic attacks.

The brain is highly sensitive to progesterone. In fact, progesterone is found in brain cells at levels twenty times higher than in the blood serum. Here, as elsewhere in the body, progesterone counterbalances the effects of estrogen. Whereas estrogen has an excitatory effect on the brain, progesterone's effect is a calming one. Women with estrogen dominance sleep restlessly, whereas progesterone replenishment enhances sleep.

The phenomenon of postpartum depression provides further evidence of the important role that progesterone plays in the brain. Keep in mind that during pregnancy, the placenta produces massive quantities of progesterone—ten to twenty times the normal amount produced in a woman's body—while the ovaries' production drops to virtually zero. After the baby is delivered, the woman's progesterone levels fall precipitously, leading to a state of estrogen dominance and functional hypothyroidism. Postpartum depression can be easily treated by taking supplemental doses of Armour Thyroid and natural, bioidentical progesterone.

Estrogen dominance is also a culprit in premenstrual headaches and migraines. One reason for this is that estrogen promotes water retention. Because the brain is confined to the fixed space of the skull, when it swells the pressure that develops causes a headache. Estrogen also causes dilation of the blood vessels. The constriction of blood vessels followed by rebound dilation is a key factor in migraines. Finally, estrogen dominance leads to depletion of the mineral magnesium, which is crucial to normal blood vessel tone. Magnesium deficiency can cause a spasm of arteries in the brain.

"Not tonight, dear ... I have a headache," is not a tired cliché. For many women in their midthirties and beyond, frequent headaches are the inevitable result of estrogen dominance. So is low libido. Sexual desire does not occur in the sexual organs—it occurs in the brain. Estrogen dominance can dampen sexual desire by increasing levels of sex hormone–binding globulins. These proteins attach to progesterone and testosterone in the bloodstream and inactivate them, just as thyroid-binding globulins do to thyroid hormones. Keep in mind that both progesterone and testosterone peak at ovulation, enhancing libido at the time when a woman is fertile. If a woman is estrogen dominant, with correspondingly high levels of sex hormone–binding globulins, she may be disinterested in sex even at the most fertile time in her cycle.

ESTROGEN DOMINANCE AND ALLERGIES

I opened this chapter by commenting on a curious relationship I had observed between the onset of allergies and changes in a woman's menstrual cycle. This relationship is no mere coincidence. Once again, estrogen dominance plays a role. Maggie, whose story opened this book, developed allergies after giving birth to her first child. Gail's allergies emerged in her midthirties, around the time that she began experiencing painful periods and other symptoms of estrogen dominance.

One explanation for the link between estrogen dominance and allergies is that estrogen promotes the release of histamine, the chemical that is responsible for troublesome allergy symptoms such as nasal congestion, watery eyes, coughing, and wheezing. Another explanation, which I'll be discussing in greater detail in the next chapter, has to do with the relationship between progesterone and the adrenal hormone cortisol. Cortisol, which is made in the adrenal glands from progesterone, is the body's natural anti-inflammatory hormone. In fact, synthetic drugs, commonly called "cortisone," are sometimes prescribed for bronchial asthma, a severe allergic condition, because they mimic the anti-inflammatory action of the body's own cortisol.

Because cortisol is made by the body from progesterone, a decline in progesterone levels will result in a decline in cortisol levels as well. It is not surprising, then, that new mothers, women in their middle years experiencing anovulatory cycles, and menopausal women whose ovaries are no longer producing progesterone may also have insufficient cortisol and begin experiencing allergies to substances that were previously innocuous to them.

Estrogen Dominance and Breast Cancer

The most serious consequence of estrogen dominance is breast cancer. As I mentioned earlier in this chapter, estrogen dominance could also be called progesterone deficiency, because it is the imbalance between estrogen and progesterone in a woman's body that causes so many physical and emotional problems at midlife. A number of studies have found that insufficient progesterone may be a more important factor than excessive estrogen in increasing a woman's risk of breast cancer.

One of the most significant studies of the relationship between low levels of natural progesterone and increased breast cancer risk was published in the *American Journal of Epidemiology* in August 1981. In this study, conducted by researchers from Johns Hopkins University's School of Public Health, women of childbearing age who were having difficulty conceiving were divided into two groups. The first group consisted of women whose infertility was attributed to progesterone deficiency, while the second group was composed of women with infertility due to nonhormonal causes. All of the women were followed for thirteen to thirty-three years and the incidence of breast cancer in each group was recorded.

At the study's conclusion, researchers found that the infertile women with progesterone deficiency had a premenopausal breast cancer risk that was 540 percent greater than that of women whose infertility was not related to their hormone status. Not only that, but these women had a 1,000 percent greater risk of death from all types of cancer. After menopause, when estrogen levels declined, the breast cancer risk was similar in the two groups, suggesting that progesterone's protective effects were much more critical during the premenopausal period.

While I would not presume to suggest that progesterone is a cure for breast cancer, this study certainly supports the theory that it can help prevent it. Other research suggests that natural, bioidentical progesterone may delay the progression of this often deadly disease. Several studies have found that topical estrogen increases the rate of cellular division of breast epithelial cells, which are the cells that can become malignant. In contrast, topical progesterone slows down this cell division.

If you are wondering why so little has been written about natural, bioidentical hormones until recently, the answer is that for almost four decades counterfeit hormones were universally embraced by the medical profession as wonder drugs. The mainstream media reinforced this image, portraying counterfeit hormone replacement therapy (HRT) as a veritable fountain of youth. The counterfeit estrogens in particular were credited with seemingly magical powers to prevent age-related maladies as varied as osteoporosis and Alzheimer's disease, colon cancer and heart disease. Negative studies, of which there were a growing number, were largely ignored by the media in favor of glowing reports that suggested female hormone replacement could enhance a woman's quality of life and extend her years. But ignoring the negative studies didn't make them go away.

WOMEN'S HEALTH INITIATIVE

For this reason, in 1993, the Women's Health Initiative (WHI) began enrolling postmenopausal women for a nationwide, long-term study of the benefits and risks of conventional HRT using the popular drug Prempro, a combination of Premarin and Provera. Once enough women had been recruited, the study was scheduled to last eight and a half years. However, it was ended abruptly three years early due to the increased risk of breast cancer in women using counterfeit hormones. The study findings, published in the *Journal of the American Medical Association* on July 17, 2002, sent shockwaves through the medical profession, the media, and the public.

The researchers reported that the risk of breast cancer increased with each year that a woman remained on HRT, so that after five years, a woman who was taking HRT had a 26 percent higher risk of breast cancer than a woman who was not using hormones. Women using counterfeit hormones also experienced significantly higher risks of coronary heart disease, stroke, and pulmonary embolism (blood clots to the lungs) than women who were not using hormones.

A year after the findings from the WHI were reported, British researchers reported equally disturbing findings from the Million Women Study, a five-year analysis of the relationship between HRT and breast cancer risk in the United Kingdom. In this study, which was published in the premier British medical journal *The Lancet* on August 9, 2003, researchers found that postmenopausal women who were current users of HRT had a 66 percent higher risk of developing breast cancer and a 22 percent higher risk of dying of breast cancer than women who had never used HRT.

Based on their findings, these researchers estimated that the use of HRT by postmenopausal women in the United Kingdom had resulted in twenty thousand extra cases of breast cancer over the preceding decade. The most dangerous HRT combination, which was responsible for 75 percent of the breast cancers, was synthetic equine (horse) estrogen (e.g., Premarin, Cenestin, and Ogen) plus progestin (counterfeit progesterone).

AN OUNCE OF PREVENTION IS WORTH A
POUND OF CURE

There has been a tremendous push for "The Cure for Breast Cancer" in this country. However, this slogan completely misses a fundamental truth about what women want. No woman wants to develop breast cancer, then submit to disfiguring, painful, or toxic therapies with the hope of being cured. Women want and deserve safe, effective measures to prevent breast cancer and the other maladies that occur during midlife.

The past quarter-century of research has clearly demonstrated that low levels of human progesterone increase the risk of breast cancer. This was the conclusion of the 1981 Johns Hopkins study that found a much higher incidence of breast cancer among women with infertility due to progesterone deficiency compared to women with infertility due to nonhormonal causes.

The WHI, Million Women Study, and other recent studies of conventional HRT, all of which have found that counterfeit hormones increase the risk of breast cancer, provide further evidence for this hypothesis. In both the WHI and the Million Women Study, the highest risk of breast cancer was associated with the use of the combination of synthetic equine estrogen plus progestin. In fact, it is likely that the progestin component was the major factor in this increased risk, because progestins turn off the ovaries' production of naturally occurring progesterone, reducing levels of this protective hormone. The use of counterfeit HRT also leads to hypothyroidism, which has been demonstrated to significantly increase the risk of cancer. This is because hypothyroidism causes a state of low oxidative metabolism, an environment in which cancer thrives.

There is a huge, multi-billion-dollar cancer industry in America. There is also a multi-billion-dollar pharmaceutical industry and a multi-billion-dollar medical industry in this country. While these highly profitable industries may pay lip service to preventive practices such as healthy eating, exercise, and smoking cessation, they will never embrace prevention as a primary strategy for reducing the death toll from cancer or any other disease. The reason is simple economics. There is no money to be made from preventing disease. Healthy people do not need surgery, drugs, or doctors.

The primary goal of medicine should be the prevention of disease rather than the treatment of disease. The old adage remains true, "An ounce of prevention is worth a pound of cure." Clearly, the first step in prevention is to refrain from using counterfeit hormones, which have been demonstrated to cause cancer rather than to prevent it.

Step two is to use bioidentical hormones. This means first and foremost bioidentical progesterone, both to reduce the risk of breast cancer and to alleviate the symptoms of estrogen dominance that occur in midlife. Progesterone supplementation should begin around the age of thirty-five or younger, whenever the symptoms of progesterone deficiency occur. Premenstrual symptoms such as breast tenderness, headaches, mood swings, depression, fluid retention, weight gain, and irregular or heavy periods are common signs of progesterone deficiency and are highly responsive to treatment with bioidentical progesterone. As women enter menopause, the addition of bioidentical estrogen may be warranted to alleviate menopausal symptoms.

A TALE OF TWO "HORMONES"

What exactly is Prempro, and why is it so harmful to a
woman's health? Prempro refers to the most popular form
of HRT, a counterfeit estrogen called Premarin combined
with a counterfeit progesterone called Provera. Premarin is
a combination of horse estrogens derived from pregnant
mares' urine (hence the name Pre + mar + in). While
this may be a fine preparation for mares in menopause,
it is of dubious benefit for human beings. Not only does
counterfeit estrogen fail to improve the quality or length of
a woman's life, it can cause serious and even fatal diseases
including endometrial cancer, breast cancer, strokes, and
life-threatening blood clots in the lungs.

And what of the counterfeit progesterone drug,
Provera? Like conjugated equine estrogens, Provera is the
invention of the pharmaceutical industry. Although its
generic name (medroxyprogesterone) makes Provera sound
like it is a form of progesterone, it is not. It is a progestin,
a drug that exists nowhere in nature. Unlike natural
progesterone, which is essential to the development of the
unborn baby, Provera can cause miscarriage or birth defects
if taken during the first four months of pregnancy. It can
also cause symptoms identical to those caused by estrogen
dominance, including breast tenderness, migraines, allergy
and asthma symptoms, weight gain, and depression. Taking
higher doses of Provera in a misguided attempt to correct
a condition of estrogen dominance won't alleviate these
symptoms, because Provera isn't natural progesterone. It's
a counterfeit hormone, and you can't fool Mother Nature.

What Does "Natural" or "Bioidentical" Mean?

I have been using the word "counterfeit" to refer to patented drug company hormonal preparations and "natural" or "bioidentical" to refer to the kinds of hormones that I and other wellness physicians recommend. I prefer the term "bioidentical" because it accurately conveys the most important aspect of these hormones. They are biologically identical to hormones produced in our bodies.

Natural, bioidentical hormones are derived from a plant molecule called diosgenin found in soybeans and wild yams. After diosgenin is extracted from these plants, it is converted into bioidentical progesterone in the laboratory. In turn, progesterone can be converted by a chemist into the three human estrogen hormones: estradiol, estrone, and estriol.

Because natural progesterone and the estrogens are biologically identical in structure to the hormones produced by the body, the cells of a woman's body respond to them in exactly the same way that they respond to the hormones produced in her own body. This is good news for women, but the fact that these bioidentical hormones cannot be patented makes them unattractive to the pharmaceutical companies. Pharmaceutical drugs can only be patented if they are chemically unique, unlike any currently existing drug and unlike any substance that exists in nature.

This is the reason that you will rarely see major drug companies producing and promoting natural hormone preparations. Drug companies derive the bulk of their billion-dollar profits from the first seventeen or so years of a drug's life, when its patent status protects it from competition and enables the company that holds the patent to charge whatever the market will bear. Without the possibility of patenting natural, bioidentical hormones, the drug companies have no incentive to produce and sell these hormones. The profit margin is just too low.

Wild Yam Cream Is Not the Same as Natural Progesterone

Many health food stores carry wild yam creams that contain the plant hormone diosgenin. While diosgenin can be converted into human-identical progesterone in a laboratory, it cannot be converted into progesterone or any other hormone in a woman's body. Wild yam creams will not yield the benefits of a bioidentical progesterone product that contains the human-identical form of this hormone.

Transdermal skin creams containing genuine USP progesterone are available without a prescription, but their strengths are low and their qualities vary widely. Some contain mineral oil, which prevents the progesterone from being readily absorbed through the skin. Others are improperly stabilized, meaning that exposure to oxygen over time will degrade the potency of the product. Still others contain insufficient dosages of progesterone to achieve any real benefits. This is why it is best to be evaluated and treated by a physician trained in the use of bioidentical hormones so that an optimal dose of progesterone can be prescribed.

The type of progesterone that I recommend and use in my practice is oral micronized slow-release progesterone in capsule form. Oral progesterone that has not been micronized is poorly absorbed by the body—only about 10 percent ends up in circulation as progesterone—and therefore extremely high doses must be taken in order to get a therapeutic dose to the cells. It is also excreted from the body very rapidly, so there is a surge in progesterone levels, followed by a dramatic drop.

These problems do not occur with oral micronized slow-release progesterone. Micronized comes from a Greek word, micron, which is a measure of length equal to one-millionth of a meter. Micronized progesterone contains extremely tiny particles, 80–90 percent of which are absorbed by the body, so that lower doses may be used. And because the hormone is released slowly, it is absorbed through the lymphatic system and the tiny capillaries of the small intestines, which allows for a steady delivery of progesterone to the cells.

NATURAL ESTROGEN: USE ONLY AS NEEDED

Not all women, even those who are menopausal or who have had a hysterectomy, need estrogen. As I hope I've made clear, many of the symptoms attributed to estrogen deficiency are actually caused by a relative excess of estrogen and are best treated with natural progesterone to restore the proper balance. In addition, even after menopause or a hysterectomy, a woman's body continues to make estrogen in her fat cells. However, for women who are experiencing hot flashes, night sweats, or vaginal dryness, bioidentical estrogen can be beneficial.

When used in conjunction with progesterone, bioidentical estrogen also may be useful for women at risk of osteoporosis. While it will not help build bone, which is the function of progesterone, the use of bioidentical estrogen can help slow bone breakdown.

Bioidentical estrogen is available only by prescription. Recall that "estrogen" is actually the name for a class of hormones. The form of bioidentical estrogen that I recommend is oral micronized bi-estrogen, called Bi-Est. Bi-Est is composed of 80 percent estriol, the least stimulating of the estrogens and the one that seems most beneficial to the vagina, cervix, and vulva, and 20 percent estradiol, the most stimulative of the estrogens. The ratio of estriol to estradiol may be varied to control symptoms.

IF MOMMA AIN'T HAPPY . . .

The old adage, "If momma ain't happy, ain't nobody happy," is really true. When a woman is suffering from a hormonal imbalance, it affects much more than her reproductive organs. It affects her mood, her energy, her outlook on life, as well as her relationships with family members, friends, and coworkers.

Louise, whose story I shared at the beginning of this chapter, had no idea of the toll that her hormonal imbalance had taken in her life and in her relationships with loved ones until the proper balance was restored. Not surprisingly, when I saw her for her follow-up visit after she had begun taking bioidentical hormones, her elation over finally feeling well was mixed with sadness and regret.

"I reflected on my life over the past twenty years," she told me, "and then wrote my son a letter apologizing for being such an irritable, moody, depressed mother. He was five years old when I had my hysterectomy. I just wish I had known about natural progesterone then."

Gail also expressed regret that she had not known about natural progesterone when she was in her twenties and thirties. A year and a half after she first consulted me, she told me that the treatment had had an unexpected dividend—it had improved her marriage. "Life is so much happier around the house. My husband has said he would pay double for all that you have done for my health."

I was pleased by the news that Gail's relationship with her husband had improved, but was not surprised. I often remind our staff that we save marriages without doing any counseling. When women achieve hormonal balance, the improvement in their health and quality of life enhances their family lives, their marital lives, their social lives, and their work lives.

It would have been so easy for me to have ignored the problems caused by hormonal imbalances that occur in so many women during midlife. But Dr. Fred had taught me the importance of asking questions, listening to what my patients had to say, and always looking for the underlying patterns in illness. As I applied this simple principle in my medical practice, patterns did indeed begin to emerge. Now all that I had to do was determine what was causing these patterns to develop. Because I was willing to accept information from my patient, Linda, concerning natural progesterone, a whole new opportunity to offer health and wellness to my patients presented itself.

Thank you, Linda!

CHAPTER 8
Testosterone: For Men, and Women Too

Among conventional physicians, the phrase "hormone replacement therapy" refers to the use of estrogen, with or without progesterone, to alleviate symptoms of menopause or to prevent or treat conditions associated with estrogen deficiency, such as heart disease and osteoporosis. What it generally does *not* refer to is the use of testosterone to prevent and treat these very same conditions, despite the well-documented role of testosterone in cardiovascular health and bone density. Nor does it refer to the use of testosterone as a therapy for the fatigue, depression, mental decline, and other symptoms of testosterone deficiency that occur with increasing age.

The failure to acknowledge that levels of testosterone decline with age and to address this deficiency is a glaring oversight on the part of conventional physicians. Although the decline in testosterone that begins in midlife is more gradual than the dramatic drop in estrogen that occurs at menopause, it nevertheless has significant effects on health and well-being—and I'm not talking exclusively about male health and well-being.

It is true that women produce much smaller amounts of testosterone even in the prime of life, but this does not mean that they are spared the effects of a decline in levels of this hormone. Let's begin by looking at the crucial role played by testosterone in the health and well-being of women.

THE DWINDLING OF FEMALE SEXUAL DESIRE

In February 1999, researchers published a report in the *Journal of the American Medical Association* entitled "Sexual Dysfunction in the United States." Using data from the National Health and Social Life Survey, a study of adult sexual behavior in the United States, they calculated the incidence of various sexual problems among adults aged 18–59. Among the women in this representative sample, the number one problem was low libido, which affected almost one-third of survey respondents.

Why are so many women uninterested in sex? There are many possible reasons, both physical and psychological. In my experience as a physician who has treated thousands of women over the years, one underappreciated explanation for a woman's loss of interest in sex is inattention by her husband or male companion—both in the bedroom and outside of it. A man who consistently performs intercourse to achieve his own pleasure, without giving attention to his wife's feelings, will usually find a passive, disinterested sexual partner.

Women are more responsive to men who understand that lovemaking is an ongoing experience of affection. A woman who is not listened to, appreciated, or gratified sexually by her husband or male companion is unlikely to be romantically inclined.

However, there is another reason why women may experience a decline in libido, especially as they pass into their thirties, forties, and beyond: a deficiency of testosterone.

If you're wondering what testosterone has to do with a woman's interest in sex, the answer is: everything. In women as well as men, testosterone is the hormone of desire. The millions of women in this country who experience estrogen dominance suffer not only from a relative deficiency of progesterone but also from a deficiency of testosterone.

As I mentioned in the previous chapter, in women who are of reproductive age, levels of testosterone peak at ovulation, the very time in a woman's menstrual cycle when she is fertile. This surge in testosterone midway through her cycle stimulates a woman's desire for sex. However, when a woman is estrogen dominant, she experiences numerous anovulatory cycles in which there is no elevation in testosterone at this midpoint. This problem is compounded by the fact that estrogen dominance increases the liver's production of sex hormone–binding globulins, proteins that attach to the small amount of testosterone in circulation and inhibit the hormone's entry into cells.

SIGNS AND SYMPTOMS OF
LOW TESTOSTERONE IN WOMEN:

- Low libido
- Blunted motivation
- Fatigue
- Depression and/or anxiety
- Low blood levels of free testosterone

If estrogen dominance is bad news for a woman's libido, a hysterectomy can be devastating. About half of a woman's testosterone is produced by her ovaries, with the other half produced in the adrenal glands. Women who undergo a total hysterectomy, with the removal of their ovaries, immediately lose 50 percent of their circulating testosterone. The resulting symptoms of low libido, fatigue, and malaise often are attributed wrongly to the sharp drop in estrogen, when in fact it is the abrupt decline in testosterone levels that is the culprit. The primary sexual effect of estrogen deficiency is thinning and dryness of the vaginal tissues, not a decrease in desire. For women who undergo natural menopause, the decline in testosterone is more gradual, but it still can dampen libido and contribute to depression, anxiety, and other psychological symptoms.

The solution is obvious: supplementation with small, physiologic replacement doses of natural testosterone to restore levels to those of a healthy young woman. Sadly, this option is rarely offered to women by conventional physicians.

As with estrogen and progesterone, the form of testosterone that I recommend for women is time-released micronized capsules. Micronized hormones are 80–90 percent absorbed, and the time-release base allows for the slow, steady absorption of testosterone in the small intestines and the lymphatic system. The dose is adjusted as necessary according to a woman's symptoms and periodic measurements of free testosterone levels in the blood, if indicated.

Besides its beneficial effects on female sexual desire and pleasure, testosterone improves the tone of the vagina and bladder, decreases body fat, improves muscle strength and bone density, enhances the function of thyroid hormone, relieves anxiety and depression, and promotes clearer thinking.

REAL MEN DO NEED TESTOSTERONE

If testosterone can do all this for women, imagine what it can do for the millions of men who experience an age-related decline in testosterone levels. After all, testosterone is the quintessential male hormone. An abundance of testosterone is not only what sets men apart from women—it is also what separates the men from the boys. The physical effects of testosterone become glaringly apparent when boys enter puberty. The surge in testosterone at this time causes a boy's voice to change from soprano to bass, hair to sprout on his face, muscles to develop on his arms, and thoughts of the opposite sex to arise with increasing frequency.

Testosterone is also responsible for differences in the structure and function of the male brain. Prenatal exposure to testosterone enlarges a region of the hypothalamus involved in male-typical sex behavior and increases the size of clusters of spinal cord neurons that serve the external genitals. As a result of higher levels of testosterone, males are more aggressive and self-confident. There are cognitive differences as well. Males consistently outperform females on tests of spatial ability and mathematics, although they do not perform as well as women on tests of verbal ability.

Much of what we know about the importance of testosterone to male sexual behavior, mood, cognition, and well-being comes from studies of men who suffer from hypogonadism, in which the testicles do not produce sufficient levels of testosterone. Due to their profound testosterone deficiency, hypogonadal men typically suffer from low libido and erectile dysfunction. The good news is that when testosterone replacement therapy is initiated, these men experience a significant improvement in their sexual desire and motivation, enjoyment of sex, and ability to achieve and maintain erections.

EFFECTS OF TESTOSTERONE IN MEN

- Causes the formation of the internal and external male sex organs
- Initiates the production of sperm by the testicles
- Enhances libido and sexual potency
- Promotes the development of muscle mass, strength, and tone
- Decreases body fat
- Promotes increased bone mass
- Stimulates the production of red blood cells by the bone marrow
- Increases metabolism by enhancing the conversion of the inactive thyroid hormone, T4, to the active thyroid hormone, T3, within the cells
- Promotes male traits such as aggressiveness, spatial and mathematical ability, enhanced well-being, and self-confidence

Mood is also affected by testosterone deficiency. Studies show that testosterone-deficient men have higher levels of depression, anxiety, and irritability, and lower levels of energy and overall well-being than men with healthy testosterone levels. Again, testosterone replacement usually reverses these changes, alleviating depression and irritability, restoring energy, and enhancing overall well-being. Research demonstrates that mental ability improves with testosterone replacement in men who are testosterone deficient. (See testosterone study in appendix I.)

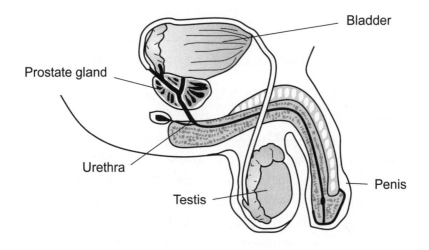

Bladder

Prostate gland

Urethra

Testis

Penis

Figure 9. The male reproductive organs.

ANDROPAUSE: THE MALE MENOPAUSE

Elderly men represent the low end of a range of testosterone values. At the other end are healthy young men in the prime of life, whose testosterone levels have reached their peak. Between these two extremes lies a continuum. The one thing we know about this continuum is that as men age, they move from a state of optimal testosterone status to one of relative deficiency. This downward slide begins in a man's thirties and continues inexorably until the day he dies.

Though not as dramatic an event as menopause, this steady, inevitable decline in testosterone is real nonetheless. And like menopause, this age-related decline in the preeminent male hormone can have a wide range of effects on the body and mind.

IS ANDROPAUSE A MODERN MALADY?

Cavemen who were fortunate to live to the "ripe old age" of forty or fifty must have suffered from a decline in testosterone levels. However, because they lived in an environment unpolluted by synthetic chemicals, it is unlikely that primitive men experienced anything like the epidemic of testosterone deficiency seen in our age.

As I mentioned in the previous chapter, petrochemicals pervade the environment and contaminate the water, air, soil, and animal and plant life. These petrochemicals are used in thousands of manufactured goods. They are found in the plastic bottles from which we drink, the chemicals used in dry cleaning, the lotions and sprays we use for personal hygiene, and the pesticides sprayed on the foods we eat, to name just a few examples.

Petrochemicals are referred to as xenoestrogens because they mimic the effects of estrogen hormones in our bodies and interfere with normal hormone function. This is a disaster for men, for not only do xenoestrogens disrupt the production of testosterone, they also antagonize the effects of testosterone in the body. Xenoestrogens are linked to the dramatic decline in the average sperm count in Western societies since the 1950s as well as to the rise in testicular cancer over the same time period. It will be years before we have the complete story on the effects of these unnatural, toxic chemicals on male fertility, health, and well-being.

As with any biological change that occurs gradually rather than abruptly, the age-related decline in testosterone often goes unnoticed until a critical point is reached. Suddenly, seemingly out of the blue, a man in his forties or fifties may begin feeling depressed, irritable, or uninterested in the things that used to give him pleasure. He may notice that he has more aches and pains and fatigues more easily. He may develop a "spare tire" around his abdomen and find that his muscles have lost their strength or tone. He may lose interest in sex, have difficulty making decisions, or experience any number of other problems related to the decline in levels of testosterone.

Though men are notoriously neglectful of their health, it is at this point that they often take action. They may begin exercising, but find that even when they work out they show little improvement in muscle strength and stamina. They may go on a diet but have trouble losing weight. The lack of progress in their fitness regimen often leaves them feeling even more discouraged.

If they consult a physician, they are most likely to be prescribed an antidepressant, as if their problem were "all in their head." But taking an antidepressant is likely to compound the problem. As in women, these drugs can cause fatigue and weight gain and are notorious for their negative effects on sexual desire and potency. At any rate, it makes no sense to prescribe a drug to treat a symptom of an underlying hormone deficiency when the deficiency itself is so easily remedied by physiologic replacement doses of natural testosterone.

WHO CAN BENEFIT FROM TESTOSTERONE REPLACEMENT?

If you are a male in your forties or older and have experienced a decline in your mood, energy, motivation, mental sharpness, sexual desire or performance, it's possible that you've entered andropause. Your testicles may not be producing enough testosterone, or you may have too little free testosterone in circulation. Keep in mind that only free testosterone is biologically active. Testosterone attached to sex hormone–binding globulin is unable to latch onto cell receptors and initiate cellular activity.

THE AGE-RELATED DECLINE IN TESTOSTERONE

Age range	Free testosterone level (pg/ml)
20–29	19–41
30–39	18–39
40–49	16–33
50–59	13–31

How can you determine if you are testosterone deficient? One way, of course, is to undergo blood testing to measure levels of free testosterone. If your level is below that considered normal for a twenty- to twenty-nine-year-old, you likely would benefit from natural testosterone replacement. However, as with female hormonal imbalance, thyroid dysfunction, and other hormonal problems, blood tests are not the be-all and end-all of diagnosis. I consider clinical symptoms to be equally if not more important, both for identifying testosterone deficiency and for evaluating the effects of treatment. After all, the goal is optimal health and wellness, not specific levels on a lab test.

Here is a list of common signs and symptoms of low testosterone that I use to determine if a man is likely to benefit from natural testosterone replacement:

SIGNS AND SYMPTOMS OF LOW TESTOSTERONE IN MEN

- Low libido
- Lack of initiative, assertiveness and drive
- Fatigue
- Decline in sense of well-being and self-confidence
- Depressed, irritable moods
- Indecisiveness
- Decreased mental sharpness
- Lessened stamina and endurance
- Loss of muscle mass, strength, and tone
- Increased body fat around the waist
- Decline in sexual ability
- Sleep apnea

Conventional physicians often warn men against the use of testosterone replacement based on a misconception that it may promote prostate cancer. Testosterone has been in use for over fifty years, and there is no evidence of such a link. In fact, it is not young men with high testosterone levels who develop prostate cancer but elderly men with low testosterone levels. Keep in mind, I am not advocating abnormally high doses of testosterone to achieve superhuman strength or aggressiveness; instead, I am recommending low-dose therapy to achieve a blood level of testosterone that is associated with optimal health and wellness.

I do recommend that men have their prostate-specific antigen (PSA) measured before beginning therapy and periodically thereafter. PSA normally rises when testosterone therapy is initiated, but it usually levels off after a few weeks. I also recommend that men take saw palmetto (160 mg twice a day). This Native American herb strengthens the prostate gland and inhibits the conversion of testosterone into its more problematic metabolite, dihydrotestosterone (DHT).

Can testosterone replacement really make a difference in a man's health and well-being? It can do that and much more. Read on to learn about a man who experienced not only improved physical and mental health but also a dramatic increase in his business when he began using natural testosterone.

RICHARD'S STORY

Richard is married, in his late fifties, and the father of two teenagers. He owns and operates a construction company that is responsible for setting up many of the major sports events and concerts in Houston, San Antonio, and other big cities in Texas. While the job is both physically strenuous and mentally taxing, Richard has always thrived on the challenges of this demanding business.

However, when Richard entered his fifties, he went into a tailspin physically and psychologically. He noticed that he had no energy and his motivation was gone. He couldn't seem to focus on anything and made some poor and costly business decisions. Normally a "take charge" kind of person, Richard now dreaded getting out of bed in the morning and avoided phone calls at the office. He began to consider selling his company and getting out of the business.

Richard consulted several physicians for help with his fatigue, lack of drive, and other problems. They weren't very helpful and didn't seem to have a clue as to what was really wrong with him. After listening to my radio program for several months, Richard decided to make an appointment to see me.

On his first visit, I sat down with Richard and asked him how he was feeling. He described his symptoms—depression, low energy, lack of motivation, trouble focusing. When I asked what the previous physicians had done to help him, he told me that the first physician he consulted had simply ordered some blood work and informed him his cholesterol was high.

"That's fine, but what does this have to do with my lack of energy and drive?" he wondered to himself as he left the office with a prescription for a cholesterol-lowering drug.

The second doctor was no better. "He just gave me a prescription antidepressant and told me to get some exercise," he said. "But that just didn't make sense. I was already getting five hours of exercise a day on the job hauling heavy equipment, working alongside my crew setting up events. I didn't see how I could get more exercise than I already was getting."

After listening to Richard's story and giving him a thorough examination, it was obvious to me that Richard was operating by sheer willpower—and there was not much willpower left. He had the classical symptoms of hypothyroidism and low testosterone. These two conditions often go hand in hand, since testosterone assists in the conversion of the inactive thyroid hormone, T4, to the active T3 form.

I explained to Richard that virtually all of his symptoms were likely related to the decline in his body's production of both testosterone and thyroid hormone. Restoring their levels to what they had been in his midtwenties would yield measurable improvements in his energy, mood, and overall well-being. Richard left the office feeling more hopeful than he had in a long time. The results of his blood tests confirmed my diagnosis and his need for thyroid and testosterone supplementation.

A month later, during a follow-up visit, Richard was positively bursting with enthusiasm. "I have improved so much mentally and physically," he said. "My energy is great, and my mental sharpness has improved 100 percent. I had no idea that I was having such trouble concentrating. The difference is remarkable!"

Richard was especially glad to have regained his passion for his business. "I was ready to sell my company," he said. "In my line of work, I have to negotiate with unions, and they are tough. I just wasn't up to it before. But now I am able to stand my ground and act decisively."

A year later, Richard continued to boast about the improvement in his health and well-being. However, he was even more elated by the benefits he had noticed in seemingly unrelated areas of his life. "In the past year, my business has tripled," he said. "I now have over four hundred employees and my income has gone up dramatically. I had no idea what an impact my health could have on my career success."

The improvement in Richard's health was what I had seen in numerous other men. It was also no surprise to me to learn of his business success. I am convinced that all wealth is founded upon good health. Richard is living proof of this.

CHAPTER 9
Stress and the Body: The Cortisol Connection

The addition of natural, bioidentical hormone therapy to my treatment regimen made a world of difference for the vast majority of my patients. But there was still a small group of patients who did not respond as expected, despite the comprehensiveness of my approach. Even with the proper balance of estrogen and progesterone, a small number of female patients still experienced menstrual irregularities, anxiety, and depression. Even when taking natural thyroid hormone, some patients with hypothyroidism continued to suffer from low energy and "brain fog." Even with allergy treatment, some patients still had recurrent sinus infections. And nearly all of them told me that they felt "stressed out."

I was frustrated by my inability to get to the root cause of these patients' health problems and asked myself, "What piece of the puzzle am I missing?" I knew there must be a common factor underlying the diverse symptoms that these patients were experiencing. Was the common factor stress, or the way their bodies responded to stress?

A SERENDIPITOUS DISCOVERY

In 1998, I learned that Dr. Broda Barnes had often prescribed natural cortisol along with Armour Thyroid. At that time, I knew little about the therapeutic use of cortisol. I knew that it was a stress hormone secreted by the adrenal glands. I knew that it had been promoted in the 1950s as a treatment for rheumatoid arthritis, but that its use had eventually been supplanted by counterfeit corticosteroids produced by the drug companies.

Like all physicians, I was aware of the potential risks of very high doses of corticosteroids, which are often prescribed for arthritis and other inflammatory conditions. However, I was not aware that very low replacement doses of the body's most important corticosteroid, cortisol, were safe and highly beneficial to patients with a wide range of symptoms.

In medical school I learned about Addison's disease, a relatively rare condition in which the adrenal gland is unable to produce adequate cortisol. But there was no mention of mild adrenal insufficiency or adrenal fatigue, its effects on immunity and on the function of other hormones, or its treatment. It was as if this condition did not exist.

I respected Dr. Barnes immensely, and since I was eager to find ways to help the patients who were not responding to my comprehensive treatment program, I decided to research the topic of natural cortisol replacement. In the fall of 1998, I purchased a medical text named, appropriately enough, *Safe Uses of Cortisol*. In this book, William McK. Jefferies, M.D., outlined the role of the adrenal glands in the body's response to stress and documented the connection between adrenal insufficiency and menstrual problems, infertility, allergies, asthma, rheumatoid arthritis, viral infections, chronic fatigue, hypothyroidism, and other ailments. Throughout the book, Dr. Jefferies presented compelling case histories from his fifty years of experience using natural cortisol.

As I read Dr. Jefferies' textbook, I became increasingly intrigued. Like my other mentors, Dr. Jefferies was a physician who challenged conventional thought. He recognized that health is a continuum from extreme disease to a condition of optimal health. Instead of assuming that only life-threatening adrenal insufficiency merited attention, he maintained that even mild adrenal insufficiency could impair health and should be treated.

Throughout his book, Dr. Jefferies made a clear-cut distinction between very high pharmacologic doses of counterfeit corticosteroids, which have severe adverse effects, and physiologic replacement doses, which safely reestablish the body's optimal levels of cortisol. He emphasized the difference between the synthetic, counterfeit corticosteroids produced by drug companies and naturally occurring cortisol produced by the body. Although he measured his patients' blood levels of cortisol, he did not rely solely on blood tests for diagnosis or treatment. He maintained, as I do, that a patient's clinical history is the best indicator of adrenal function.

THE ADRENAL GLANDS: TWO ORGANS IN ONE

The two adrenal glands, which derive their name from their location in the body ("ad" means *near*, "renal" means *kidney*), are key players in your body's response to stress. Situated on top of the kidneys, these pyramid-shaped organs, the size of walnuts, are actually two endocrine glands in one: an inner medulla, which orchestrates your short-term stress response, and an outer cortex, which mediates your adaptation to chronic stress.

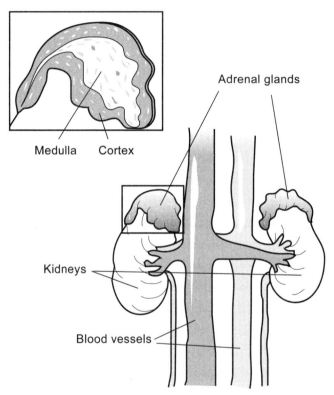

Figure 10. The adrenal glands.

The pyramid-shaped adrenal glands rest on top of the kidneys. The inner medulla secretes a short-acting hormone called epinephrine (adrenalin), while the outer cortex secretes cortisol, a hormone with more prolonged effects.

The primary hormone of the medulla is epinephrine, also called adrenalin. This powerful, short-acting hormone is secreted in response to the four *E*'s: exercise, excitement, embarrassment, and emergency. The flood of adrenaline that is unleashed in these situations causes a number of dramatic physical changes throughout your body: your heart beats more rapidly and forcefully; your pupils dilate; and blood is shunted toward your skeletal muscles, heart, and brain. Glycogen in your liver is converted into glucose to be used for quick energy. You may break out into a cold sweat and begin breathing more rapidly. In short, your body is mobilized for action. This is why adrenaline is known as the "fight or flight" hormone.

Adrenaline's effects are dramatic and unmistakable, but because this hormone does not linger in your body, its effects are also relatively short-lived. On the other hand, cortisol, the stress hormone produced by the outer cortex, has more prolonged effects on your body. If adrenaline is like the whip that drives the horse faster and faster, cortisol is like the rider's boot, digging into the flank, keeping the horse going even when it's ready to quit.

The primary function of cortisol is to promote gluconeogenesis, the conversion of fats and proteins to sugar (glucose). Gluconeogenesis is an essential component of your body's adaptation to chronic stress, ensuring that your vital organs, especially your brain, heart, and skeletal muscles, have enough energy to meet the increasing workload. In addition, cortisol assists adrenaline in stimulating the cardiovascular system, increasing the heart rate and pumping capacity and temporarily raising blood pressure. Cortisol also decreases inflammation, which is why this hormone and its counterfeit derivatives have been used to treat inflammatory conditions, such as allergies, asthma, arthritis, and skin disorders.

Due to its metabolic effects, high levels of cortisol can be extremely damaging. People with chronically elevated levels of cortisol may have high blood sugar and insulin levels and high blood pressure; they may gain weight, especially around the abdomen; and they have a greater risk of heart disease. However, just because high levels of cortisol are harmful doesn't mean that low levels are healthy. As with all hormones, balance is the key.

ADRENAL FATIGUE: A FAILURE TO ADAPT

Cortisol is essential to life. Laboratory animals that have had their adrenal glands removed can no longer produce cortisol, and they are very fragile creatures. They can function reasonably well if their environment is kept perfectly stable. However, even the slightest variation in their environment—a drop in room temperature, for example—can spell death for these creatures. With the loss of their adrenal glands, they have lost their ability to adapt.

Human beings are not laboratory animals, and the environments we live in are seldom stable. We are exposed to a constant onslaught of stressors—noise, pollution, traffic, inclement weather, injuries, illnesses, emotional conflicts, deadlines, and on and on. We may heap stress on top of stress by smoking, eating refined carbohydrates, drinking coffee, or going without adequate sleep. Chronic, unrelenting stress, whether physical or psychological or both, eventually leads to adrenal fatigue. The adrenals simply cannot produce enough cortisol to meet the demands. The result? We feel "stressed out"—because we are.

As you might expect, some of the effects of suboptimal cortisol levels are the opposite of those seen with high cortisol levels. Instead of hyperglycemia, or elevated blood sugar, individuals with mild adrenal fatigue often have hypoglycemia, or low blood sugar. Instead of high blood pressure, they may have low blood pressure. Instead of feeling mentally stimulated, they may have trouble concentrating. But the number one symptom of adrenal insufficiency is fatigue. Whereas individuals with optimal cortisol levels have energy to burn, those with low cortisol levels drag themselves through the day, feeling exhausted.

If you have adrenal fatigue, you may function reasonably well when your life is stable but fall apart if stress is added. You are likely to be more vulnerable to infections and to heal more slowly than those with healthy adrenal glands. You may suffer from headaches, heart palpitations, or joint and muscle pain. You may develop allergies or chemical sensitivities or experience a worsening of existing allergies or asthma.

SYMPTOMS AND SIGNS OF ADRENAL FATIGUE

- Chronic fatigue
- Low blood sugar (hypoglycemia)
- Low blood pressure (hypotension)
- Dizziness or lightheadedness upon standing
- Muscle and/or joint pain
- Recurrent infections
- Allergies and/or asthma
- Irregular menstrual cycles
- Infertility
- Low libido
- Headaches
- Hair loss
- Dry skin
- Anxiety or panic attacks
- Depression
- Heart palpitations
- Difficulty "bouncing back" from stress
- Cold and heat intolerance

If you think that many of these symptoms sound similar to those of hypothyroidism, you're right. Although they are clinically distinct conditions, adrenal insufficiency and hypothyroidism are both metabolic problems that result in a slowdown of the body's functions and a decline in energy. Some people have only one of these conditions, but many people have both. If your hypothyroidism is complicated by adrenal insufficiency, then it's important to address this underlying problem at the same time. Let me explain why.

THE ADRENAL GLANDS AND THE THYROID: PARTNERS IN HEALTH

As I mentioned at the beginning of this chapter, some patients with hypothyroidism do not regain their energy even when they are taking natural thyroid. I was puzzled by this phenomenon until I learned about Dr. Barnes's use of natural cortisol and read Dr. Jefferies' book. Dr. Jefferies had found that adrenal fatigue often occurs in conjunction with hypothyroidism, and that, in the absence of adequate cortisol, thyroid hormone replacement was less effective.

The reason is that when the adrenal glands are weak, even normal thyroid activity is a burden. Adding supplemental thyroid hormone may result in initial improvement in energy levels and other symptoms, but as the adrenal glands become more exhausted, energy production is shut down. The solution is not more thyroid hormone. What is called for is adrenal support with small doses of cortisol.

In my experience, as well as that of Drs. Jefferies and Barnes, low-dose cortisol can make a tremendous difference in the energy and well-being of patients with hypothyroidism. Not only does it improve energy, raise body temperature, and increase resistance to infection, it also helps the body utilize thyroid hormone. Natural cortisol is especially helpful for patients with autoimmune thyroiditis, an extremely common cause of hypothyroidism that I discussed in chapter 6. Like other autoimmune conditions, autoimmune thyroiditis can develop when the adrenal glands are stressed, especially following pregnancy or at menopause. As documented in Dr. Jefferies' book, natural cortisol actually reduces levels of thyroid antibodies, enhancing the effectiveness of thyroid hormone.

ADRENAL FATIGUE AND WOMEN

Like hypothyroidism, adrenal fatigue affects women much more frequently than men. The reason women develop estrogen dominance is discussed in chapter 1. High levels of estrogen cause a corresponding increase in levels of cortisol-binding globulin. Like other hormone-binding globulins, cortisol-binding globulin interferes with hormone function. It circulates in the bloodstream, binds to cortisol, and renders it inactive. A woman with estrogen dominance may have adequate levels of total cortisol in her bloodstream, but her free, available cortisol level may be very low. Only free cortisol can pass through cell membranes and activate receptors inside the cell.

Estrogen impairs adrenal function in another way: it interferes with the release of cortisol from the adrenal cortex. In laboratory animals, when estrogen levels are high, the adrenal cortex fails to respond to signals from the brain. In other words, even though the brain is emitting a cry of alarm—"Send more cortisol!"—the gland responsible for meeting this demand does not "receive" it.

Just as estrogen dominance can contribute to adrenal insufficiency, adrenal insufficiency can contribute to estrogen dominance. Cortisol is made in the adrenal cortex from progesterone. If progesterone levels are low, then cortisol levels are likely to be low as well. Because the body considers cortisol more important to survival than progesterone, whatever progesterone is available in the adrenal cortex is going to be converted into cortisol. This means that a woman whose ovaries are producing less progesterone will not be able to call upon her adrenal glands to produce adequate amounts of cortisol.

As we age, our adrenal glands produce less cortisol. This inevitebly leads to adrenal fatigue to one degree or another.

ADRENAL FATIGUE AND ALLERGIES

Adrenal fatigue is also a common underlying problem in patients with allergies, especially when these allergies have been poorly managed. As I explained in chapter 4, out-of-control allergies often lead to recurrent sinus infections, which lead to repeated courses of antibiotic therapy, which lead to yeast overgrowth and impaired immunity. This cycle of infection, antibiotic treatment, impaired immunity, and reinfection adds stress to the body, weakening the adrenals, and reducing cortisol levels.

This in turn worsens allergies, because cortisol is the body's antiallergy hormone of choice. Cortisol is both a natural antihistamine and a natural anti-inflammatory. Prednisone, dexamethasone, and other high-dose counterfeit corticosteroids that are used to alleviate the inflammation of bronchial asthma, rheumatoid arthritis, and other autoimmune conditions are simply the drug companies' counterfeit versions of the body's own natural anti-inflammatory hormone, cortisol.

Though I don't prescribe cortisol to every patient with allergies, I have found that those with long-standing, unmanaged allergies are usually suffering from adrenal fatigue. The addition of cortisol to their treatment regimen lessens the likelihood of recurrent sinus infections and helps them regain energy more quickly.

THE IMPORTANCE OF ADRENAL SUPPORT

The use of physiologic, subreplacement doses of cortisol has proven to be a godsend for many of my patients with these and other conditions. A young, healthy person produces 20–30 mg of cortisol per day. My starting dose of slow-release biologically identical cortisol is 1.25–2.5 mg per day, and I adjust the dosage incrementally as symptoms warrant. Along with this, I also recommend that patients take dehydroepiandrosterone (DHEA), another hormone produced by the adrenal glands. The amount of DHEA produced by the adrenal cortex is greater than that of any of the other adrenal hormones, including the androgens (androstenedione and testosterone) and the estrogens (estradiol, estrone, and estriol).

Levels of DHEA and its derivative, DHEAS, peak in young adulthood and then begin to decline. By the age of seventy, your DHEA level may be less than a fifth of what it was at the age of twenty. In elderly adults, higher levels of DHEA correspond with better health and longevity. When blood levels are low, supplemental DHEA often enhances energy, immunity, and libido.

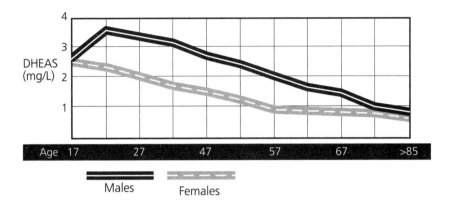

Figure 11. Age-related decline in DHEAS.
Levels of DHEAS, a blood marker of DHEA status, peak around
age seventeen in women and age twenty-two in men. After the age of thirty,
levels of DHEAS decline about 2 percent per year.

A healthy diet is also important for anyone with adrenal insufficiency. If low blood sugar is a problem, you may find it helpful to eat several small meals during the day. Make sure to include adequate protein and reduce or eliminate refined carbohydrates, caffeine, and alcohol, all of which stress the adrenal glands.

Nutritional supplements are also vital. You can find more on this important topic in appendix C, but for now, I want to mention one nutrient in particular that is crucial to healthy adrenal glands: vitamin C. The adrenal cortex has the highest concentration of vitamin C of all the organs in the body, and the cells of this gland use it at a higher rate than any other cells. Vitamin C enhances immunity, which is often impaired in those with adrenal insufficiency. During times of stress, our bodies excrete vitamin C more rapidly, making our need for this vitamin even greater.

I advise all of my adult patients to supplement with 3,000–6,000 mg of vitamin C per day. A slow-release buffered form is best to prevent overacidity of the stomach and to ensure sustained blood levels throughout the day.

CAN STRESS BE A GOOD THING?

Hans Selye, M.D., the endocrinologist who is considered the father of modern stress research, said: "I cannot and should not be cured of my stress, but merely taught to enjoy it."

There is simply no avoiding physical and psychological stress in our daily lives. If we're fortunate, the amount of stress in our lives is manageable, and if we're very fortunate, our lives include just the right amount of "good stress." Good stress is the kind of stress that brings out the best in us. It stimulates us to perform at a higher level.

Maybe the following example will help you understand what I mean. The Christmas season can be stressful; planning for parties, purchasing and wrapping gifts, decorating and making the home ready for guests, preparing meals, and entertaining relatives. But many women find the experience gratifying. This is good stress, and it allows them to bring out nurturing aspects of their personalities.

Too much stress can be overwhelming to both the body and the soul, but too little stress can be "underwhelming," resulting in boredom and a lack of vital energy. While I would never wish harmful stress—distress—upon anyone, I do encourage you to find sources of good stress in your life. Seek out activities that challenge your mind, engage your senses, and make you feel more alive. This is the kind of stress that will keep you young and make your life exhilarating.

FATHER KNEW BEST

As you mature, you will need activities and responsibilities that keep you mentally alert and physically healthy. My dad preached this and practiced it.

When my father was in his midsixties he told me, "I have no plans of retiring. Every one of my friends who has retired has died within a few years or is in some nursing home or retirement center. I love where I am in life: I am the leader of my businesses and a valuable contributor to our family. I love working with your brothers; I enjoy my friends in the oil and gas industry; I enjoy building our family business. No, I'll never retire. I plan on dying right here at CECO."

Fifteen productive years later, Dad died on the job at the age of eighty.

The night before he died, I had called my dad and asked him how he was doing. He answered, "I haven't felt this good since I was a teenager."

Dad lived a full, rich, involved, and meaningful life until the day he died. He shared his life and wealth with others. He always had a positive, upbeat attitude and saw the potential in everyone he met. Dad loved his work and viewed it as an opportunity to help others solve their problems. Dad never tried to impress anyone. He made everyone around him feel comfortable and appreciated.

Dad had always been very successful, but he was even more so in his seventies. These were his most productive years. He enjoyed the good stress of maintaining responsibility for leading his family and businesses and making things happen.

Dad set a super example for all of us.

Chapter 10

What Is the Ideal Diet?

In 1998, I attended the annual conference of the Broda O. Barnes Research Foundation, an organization dedicated to research and education in thyroid disorders. One of the guest speakers at that conference was Barry Sears, Ph.D., who had recently published a best-selling nutrition book called *The Zone: A Dietary Road Map*. Dr. Sears discussed the intimate connection between the foods we eat, our hormone levels, and our overall health and well-being.

Dr. Sears, who held a Ph.D. in biochemistry, had become a dietary expert out of personal necessity. His grandfather, father, and three uncles had all suffered fatal heart attacks before the age of fifty-four. He was convinced that, unless he found a way to defuse his "genetic time bomb," he would succumb to a similar fate.

As a chemist, Dr. Sears was an expert in manipulating molecules to achieve specific effects. His ambition was to synthesize a drug that would act like a biochemical Roto-Rooter, clearing out the cholesterol-laden plaques that are at the core of heart disease. The bad news, at least for his dream of becoming a pharmaceutical tycoon, is that his search for an "anti-atherosclerosis" drug was unsuccessful. The good news is that he found a much simpler and more palatable way to defeat heart disease: food.

But the best news of all is that the eating plan formulated by Dr. Sears is much more than a diet to prevent heart disease. It is a lifelong eating plan for anyone who wants to lose fat, gain energy, slow the aging process, and enjoy optimal health and well-being.

It is, incidentally, an eating plan that runs counter to what the U.S. government has been recommending for over two decades.

GOVERNMENT-SANCTIONED GRAINS

For over twenty-five years, the U.S. government has been telling Americans to eat less fat and more carbohydrates. It started in 1977, when a Senate committee published a document called "Dietary Goals for the United States" that urged Americans to curb their fat intake. In 1984, the National Institutes of Health chimed in with an official recommendation that Americans eat less fat. And in 1992, the U.S. Department of Agriculture (USDA) added a third voice to the chorus when it rolled out its model of the ideal diet: the low-fat, high-carbohydrate Food Guide Pyramid.

The Food Guide Pyramid, wide at the base (grains) and narrow at the top (fats, oils, and sweets), was not the first government-sanctioned model of the ideal diet. In 1956, the USDA had given us the Basic Four food groups: meat, dairy, grains, and fruits/vegetables. In principle, the Basic Four, a square divided into four quadrants, was supposed to represent a perfectly balanced diet. Ultimately this diet was blamed for the rising incidence of heart disease. The Food Guide Pyramid was intended to reverse this trend by downplaying high-fat meat and dairy products, while giving greater importance to low-fat, high-carbohydrate grains like bread, cereal, rice, and pasta.

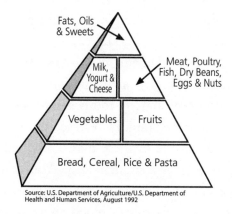

Source: U.S. Department of Agriculture/U.S. Department of
Health and Human Services, August 1992

Figure 12. USDA Food Guide Pyramid.

❈

A LEANING TOWER OF PIZZA

Starchy carbohydrates are the foundation of the USDA Food Guide Pyramid. The recommended number of servings of grains is two times the recommended number of servings of vegetables and three times the recommended number of servings of fruits, dairy products, and protein-rich animal and plant foods. While this eating plan may be a carbohydrate lover's dream, it has turned into a nutritional nightmare. In the last twenty years, our consumption of grains has increased by sixty pounds per person per year. As our intake of refined carbohydrates has ballooned, our waistlines have followed suit. We now take in up to four hundred more calories per day than we did a quarter-century ago, when the U.S. government first started recommending a low-fat diet. Not surprisingly, we are fatter than ever. Over half of all women, almost two-thirds of men, and a quarter of all children in the United States are overweight or obese. Additionally, the high carbohydrate diet has resulted in a doubling of the incidence of diabetes between 1980 and 2002.

The epidemic of diabetes in our country is not surprising once you examine the facts about grains and starches. Potatoes, bread, rice, and other starchy foods are composed of chains of simple sugars that are rapidly released into the bloodstream. Every time you eat one of these high-carbohydrate foods, your blood sugar undergoes a sudden surge. Your pancreas responds by secreting insulin, which moves glucose out of the bloodstream and into the cells. This causes blood sugar to drop, often to a level even lower than it was before you ate. In the short term, the result is reactive hypoglycemia, or low blood sugar, characterized by headache, nausea, fatigue, mental confusion, and hunger. In the long term, this roller coaster ride, with its sugar highs and sugar lows, stresses the pancreas and adrenal glands, keeps insulin levels chronically elevated, promotes weight gain, and increases your risk of not only diabetes, but also high blood pressure, heart disease, and other degenerative diseases.

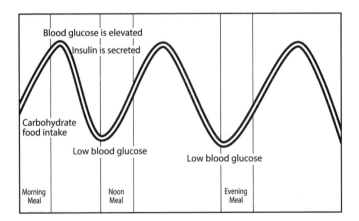

Figure 13. Reactive hypoglycemia.

A high-carbohydrate meal causes a dramatic rise in blood sugar, followed by an equally dramatic fall. This drop in blood sugar, called reactive hypoglycemia, triggers physical and mental discomfort and increases hunger. Eating more carbohydrates to satisfy hunger perpetuates this cycle.

FOOD IS MEDICINE

Clearly, food is more than just something that tastes good and satisfies your hunger. Depending on the choices you make on a day-by-day and even a meal-by-meal basis, food is something that can fuel your appetite for life or drain you of vitality.

Hippocrates, the Greek physician and founder of medicine, wrote, "Let food be your medicine and let medicine be your food." Although he lived some five hundred years before Christ, his words still ring true. Unfortunately, physicians today give only lip service to the medicinal properties of wholesome foods. The reason is simple. Most doctors learn little about nutrition in medical school beyond the basics of carbohydrate, protein, and fat metabolism. Nutrition is typically dismissed as "soft science," unworthy of serious scrutiny, while the drugs of the pharmaceutical industry are presented as the most powerful tools for preventing and curing disease. But I have yet to encounter a disease that was caused by a lack of prescription drugs. On the other hand, many diseases are caused by too few of the right foods and too many of the wrong ones.

"Let food be your medicine and let medicine be your food."

—Hippocrates, the father of medicine

A nutritionally balanced eating plan, with the right types and proportions of carbohydrates, fats, and proteins, can be your meal ticket to optimal health and wellness, which is the goal. The eating program that I recommend will lower your insulin levels, helping you to maintain a consistently high energy level by preventing blood sugar highs and lows. In the long term, it will help prevent obesity, high blood pressure, high cholesterol, diabetes, and heart disease.

HEALTHY EATING SIMPLIFIED

There is a healthy food pyramid that I promote to my patients. It minimizes the starchy, simple carbohydrates such as breads, grains, potatoes, and rice. This eating program emphasizes fiber-rich vegetables and fruits, followed by protein from low-fat meat, poultry, fish, and legumes, and small amounts of healthful fats. This is an eating plan designed to keep blood sugar levels stable.

Following this diet is not complicated. Simply eat three meals a day, and make sure that you balance your protein and carbohydrate intake at every meal. Divide your plate into three sections. The first section should contain protein, the second should contain vegetables and the third should consist of fruit. Each portion should be the no larger than the size of your fist. The protein should be eaten first, because this will help curb your cravings for carbohydrates.

Include some healthy fats from olives, nuts, or avocados, and be sure to drink a full glass of water before every meal.

As you can see, healthy eating is really very simple.

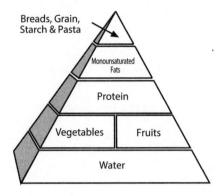

Figure 14. The balanced food pyramid.

If you want a more thorough explanation of why this eating program works, then be sure to peruse appendix B. Some suggested meal plans and recipes are also included in appendices D and E.

Bon appetit!

CHAPTER 11

Nutritional Supplements:
Your Best Form of Health Insurance

Most physicians are uneducated about the benefits of nutritional supplements. They dismiss the value of supplemental vitamins and minerals, and behave condescendingly toward their patients who use them. What a person is not up on, they are usually down on. Doctors are no different.

When I graduated from medical school in 1976, I, too, was poorly educated about the benefits of vitamins and minerals. Like most physicians, my medical education had contained at most a few lectures on the role of vitamins and minerals in the body. The vitamin deficiency diseases such as scurvy and rickets were mentioned briefly, but the effects of subclinical nutritional deficiencies were given no attention at all. Although books by nutritionist Adelle Davis were very popular among the public, they were looked down upon by conventional physicians. The notion that vitamins, minerals, and other naturally occurring substances could be used therapeutically was considered quackery.

Because I had been thoroughly indoctrinated into this mindset, I had little interest in exploring the therapeutic benefits of nutritional supplements for the first dozen years of my medical career. All that changed when my father suffered a surgical catastrophe in 1988. As I mentioned in chapter 3, my father was undergoing an angioplasty when the main artery to his heart was ruptured during the procedure. He immediately underwent emergency coronary artery bypass surgery.

Subsequently, he developed congestive heart failure, a condition in which the diseased heart greatly enlarges to compensate for its loss of muscle strength.

MY FATHER'S REQUEST

A few weeks after his surgery, my father handed me a newsletter by Julian Whitaker, M.D. This newsletter was my first encounter with the writings of Dr. Whitaker, whose monograph on natural hormones would cross my desk several years later and spur me to add biologically identical female hormones to my treatment regimen.

The topic of the newsletter my father showed me was coronary artery disease. Dr. Whitaker advised against invasive diagnostic procedures and surgery after a heart attack, citing research demonstrating that patients who underwent bypass surgery and angioplasty following a heart attack fared worse than those who were treated with prescription drugs.

Dr. Whitaker was not advocating drugs. Instead, he recommended a program of vitamin and mineral supplementation, a nutritionally balanced eating program, and exercise.

"He recommends that I take vitamins and minerals. What should I take?" asked my father.

"Dad, what the heck do I know about vitamins? I'm a doctor."

My father's eyes pierced mine as he asked, "Will you find out?"

Thus began my education in the therapeutic benefits of vitamins, minerals, amino acids, herbs, and other nutritional supplements. It is an education that continues, because new discoveries are being made every day about how these natural substances can be used to prevent and treat illness. A quick check of PubMed, the National Library of Medicine's database of peer-reviewed medical journals, reveals that in 2003 alone there were over thirteen hundred articles published on vitamin C and almost a thousand articles published on vitamin E.

Given that entire books have been written about nutritional supplements, it is difficult to do justice to this topic within the space of just one chapter. My goal here is not to tell you everything about vitamins and minerals from *A* to zinc, but to explain why a high-potency multivitamin and mineral supplement is the best health insurance policy you can buy. I will also highlight key benefits of specific vitamins and minerals and tell you how to choose a high-quality nutritional supplement.

WHO NEEDS NUTRITIONAL SUPPLEMENTS?

If you are wondering who needs nutritional supplements in a society where food is so abundant and inexpensive, the answer is: everyone. The typical American diet is high in calories but low in nutritional quality. Seventy percent of the food we eat is processed, meaning that it is stripped of essential fiber and nutrients, chemically altered, and loaded with preservatives. We eat few fresh foods and even fewer foods classified as organic, and our intake of the most nutrient-dense fruits and vegetables is abysmal. Nutrition surveys have found that, on a typical day, less than a quarter of Americans eat any vitamin-C rich foods, and less than a fifth eat broccoli, cabbage, or other cruciferous vegetables.

However, even those of us who make an effort to consume fresh fruits and vegetables are not reaping the same nutritional benefits our ancestors did. The reason? Modern agricultural methods deplete the soil of minerals, which translates to nutrient-depleted produce. Furthermore, nutrients are lost as produce is shipped from farms to grocery stores, during the cooking process, and even by being exposed to air and light.

Because our foods are nutritionally lacking, our bodies suffer, too. Studies have shown that nutritional deficiencies are surprisingly common in this country, even in apparently healthy adults.

OVER-THE-COUNTER AND PRESCRIPTION DRUGS
DEPLETE NUTRIENTS

Nearly everyone has taken an aspirin or antacid at one time or another. While these drugs may help to relieve a headache or soothe a bad case of heartburn, the downside is that they can also reduce the body's stores of certain vitamins and minerals. Regular use of aspirin can cause your folic acid levels to plummet and may interfere with the ability of vitamin C to enter cells. Frequent use of aluminum-based antacids can leach calcium from your body, increasing your risk of osteoporosis, and can inactivate vitamin B_1 (thiamine).

Prescription drugs can have even more profound effects on your body's vitamin and mineral stores, especially when they are taken for weeks, months, or years in succession. Here are just a few examples:

- Counterfeit female hormones deplete levels of vitamin B_6 and folic acid, nutrients that play an important role in reducing risk of heart disease. Not surprisingly, recent research has shown that rather than protecting women from heart disease, counterfeit female hormones actually increase heart disease risk.

- Corticosteroids are another class of drugs that cause levels of vitamin B_6 and folic acid to decline. Even more serious, these drugs can increase the risk of osteoporosis because they deplete the body of vitamin D and interfere with calcium absorption.

- Diuretics cause the loss of potassium, magnesium, zinc, and vitamin B_2. Though some diuretics "spare" potassium, they do not protect against the loss of the other important minerals and vitamins.

- The statins are cholesterol lowering drugs but they deplete the body's stores of coenzyme Q10, a compound that is essential to energy production, especially in the heart. Ironically, these drugs, which are prescribed to millions of Americans to reduce the risk of heart attack, may contribute to congestive heart failure due to their harmful effects on CoQ10 levels.

The fact is that most prescription drugs have negative effects on nutrient levels, and few doctors or patients are aware of these effects. The informational insert that you are given at the pharmacy when you pick up your prescription probably will not list nutritional deficiencies among the side effects. Yet these nutritional deficiencies may actually be the cause of fatigue, weakness, and other side effects that *are* listed, especially with drugs that are intended for long-term use. This is why taking a high-potency vitamin and mineral supplement is sound preventive medicine.

SICKNESS TAKES A TOLL ON NUTRIENT STORES

I began delving into the literature on nutritional supplements around the same time that I began my practice as an allergist. The timing couldn't have been better. I discovered that nutritional deficiencies are often an underlying factor in allergies and asthma. Correcting these nutritional deficiencies is essential to reducing the hyperreactivity of the immune system and minimizing attacks.

In fact, almost any chronic illness will drain your body's reserves of essential nutrients. This is especially likely for diseases that affect the digestion, absorption, or metabolism of nutrients, such as diabetes or inflammatory bowel disease. But even run-of-the-mill ailments like colds and sinus infections can send levels of certain nutrients into the gutter. Vitamin C and vitamin A stores can plummet during infections. And if you're prescribed an antibiotic for an infection, you may suffer additional nutrient losses, especially of B vitamins and minerals.

RDA = Ridiculously Deficient Amount

The Recommended Daily Allowances (RDAs) are like the minimum wage: barely enough to make a living and certainly not enough to ensure a high quality of life. That should not surprise you once you realize that the RDAs, which have been issued by the Food and Nutrition Board of the National Academy of Sciences since 1941, were never intended as guidelines for optimal health. The RDAs were designed to prevent serious deficiency diseases like scurvy and rickets.

In reading this book, the prevention of scurvy or rickets is probably the least of your concerns. You want to experience optimal health, not merely the absence of a deficiency disease. You want to keep your immune system in tip-top shape, possess abundant energy, and reduce your risk of diseases that pose a real threat to your quality of life such as heart disease, cancer, diabetes, arthritis, and other scourges of modern life. If this is your goal, research has shown that you'll need levels well above the RDA to promote optimal health and wellness.

In order to add years to your life and life to your years, you should take a quality nutritional supplement with high doses of antioxidants, the full range of B complex vitamins, and all of the essential minerals from calcium to zinc.

How to Choose a High-Quality Nutritional Supplement

There are a few rules of thumb that will help you identify high-quality products. First, read the label and rule out products that contain artificial colors and sweeteners, as well as wheat, corn, yeast, and other allergens.

Next, make sure that the vitamin E in your multivitamin is natural rather than synthetic. For most vitamins, it makes no difference whether the nutrient is synthesized in the lab or derived from natural sources—but this isn't true for vitamin E. Natural and synthetic vitamin E are mirror images of each other. Your body readily recognizes natural vitamin E (labeled as *d*-alpha-tocopherol), but not the synthetic form (labeled as *dl*-alpha-tocopherol). In fact, research suggests that the *l*-form may interfere with the entry of the natural *d*-form into cells.

Third, look for a product that contains minerals in chelated forms. Minerals are chelated when they are bound to an amino acid carrier, much the way they appear in foods that contain them. Examples of chelated minerals include magnesium citrate, potassium aspartate, and calcium gluconate, as well as any mineral listed as an "amino acid chelate." Research shows that chelated minerals are much more readily absorbed from the digestive tract than unchelated minerals.

Finally, check the label or product packaging for information about quality control testing. In-house quality control testing is good, while independent quality control testing is even better. If a product is formulated according to the Good Manufacturing Practices of the National Nutritional Foods Association, that's an assurance that the product meets the highest industry standards for potency and purity. And if it comes with an unconditional guarantee, you know that the company stands 100 percent behind its products.

My nutritional supplement company was founded to ensure that my patients had access to the highest-quality vitamins, minerals, herbs, amino acids, and other natural elements to promote optimal health and wellness. I put a lot of thought into my multivitamin and mineral supplement, which contains therapeutic doses of all of the key vitamins and minerals, along with other important natural compounds.

There are other conscientious manufacturers who offer high-quality nutritional supplements. Do not be overwhelmed by all of the different brands and products available. Start with a high-potency multivitamin and mineral supplement. Choose a brand in which you have confidence and take it daily. This is a wise way in which to invest in your health. All wealth is founded on health and a comprehensive nutritional supplementation program should be the cornerstone of that foundation.

For a more thorough discussion of specific vitamins, minerals and nutrients, please review the information contained in appendix C.

CHAPTER 12

Herd Mentality and the Stampede

When I opened the doors of the Hotze Health & Wellness Center, health maintenance organizations (HMOs) were in their infancy. The term "managed care" says a lot about what the insurance companies had in mind, cutting their costs by controlling the care physicians offered to their patients.

In the late 1980s, when HMOs were making their initial foray into Houston, a young representative for one of these companies pitched me on joining their plan. As he explained the scheme to me, he commented that his HMO would provide medical care for its customers.

At this point I interrupted him, pointing out what seemed to be an obvious fact. "Insurance companies don't provide medical care," I said. "Physicians do." This startled him and threw him off balance in his presentation. As he resumed his explanation of the funding mechanism, it became obvious to me that participating in HMOs would make me a lackey for the insurance companies. With my tolerance diminishing by the minute, I thanked him for his time and ended the meeting.

Are You Being Served?

You may belong to an HMO and wonder why your physician and his staff treat their patients like a herd of cattle. Let me explain how this faulty system works.

A physician who enrolls in an HMO is paid an average of five dollars per patient per month for the patients in the HMO who choose him. The physician receives this money whether or not the patient is seen. The patient often has a co-pay of ten dollars or so per visit. Now, if the physician can get paid for not seeing you, then why would he want you to have an appointment with him? The amount per year that he is paid to see you will not even cover his overhead costs.

Is it any surprise that when an HMO patient calls a physician's office to schedule an appointment, the next available opening usually is not for several weeks? Long waits and poor service discourage HMO patients from visiting the physician's office. The doctor's staff is sometimes even instructed to postpone scheduling HMO patients so that there will be openings for patients who can pay cash for their treatment.

There is no incentive for the HMO physician to provide you with excellent customer service because HMOs are all about cost cutting. HMO physicians are essentially employees of the insurance company and must follow the insurance company's policies, which limit the medical tests, procedures, and drugs that can be prescribed. If the physician controls his costs by limiting testing, then he is rewarded with a bonus at the end of the year by the insurance company.

From the beginning, I felt strongly that managed care was not in my patients' best interests and persisted in refusing to join these programs. However, the infiltration of HMOs in the Houston area continued to increase. By 1993, more and more of my established patients were enrolling in HMOs and requesting that I join them as a provider. My chief of staff at the time warned me that I would no longer be able to practice medicine unless I signed on to the HMO plans.

Thank God that my front office manager at that time, Monica Luedecke, voiced her strong opposition to this idea.

Monica had previously worked for a multidoctor pediatric practice and had experienced firsthand the administrative nightmare of managed care programs. Numerous new staff members had been hired to handle the enormous paperwork and precertification phone calls. The doctors' reimbursements had been slashed, requiring each pediatrician to see as many as eighty patients per day to make ends meet. Each time slot was double-booked, leading to extremely long waiting times for the patients and rushed office visits, lasting only a few minutes. The staff was harried and irritable. Needless to say, it was not a healthy work environment. Nor was it an environment conducive to helping patients get well.

Monica said she knew me well enough to know that I would never tolerate being required to obtain authorization from an insurance clerk to order a test, perform a procedure or initiate a treatment that both the patient and I had already decided was necessary. She told me that if I participated in these plans, I would have to slash the amount of time I spent with each patient in order to handle the increased patient volume. Finally, she reminded me that insurance companies would not allow me to offer safe and natural medical therapies but instead would force me to return to the use of drugs as the solution to my patients' problems.

As I contemplated what Monica said, the advice my mother had given me years ago came to mind: "Never follow the crowd because it is usually going in the wrong direction. Move away from the crowd and lead it in the right direction."

Monica's words, echoing those of my mother, gave me the confidence to resist the temptation to join the managed-care bandwagon. I knew in my heart that, no matter what it cost me, I had to continue to pursue the path that was leading me away from the medical mainstream, because this was the path that was helping my patients. Instead of treating my patients' symptoms with drugs, which often had side effects that required more drugs, I was committed to pursuing the path that enabled me to treat the root cause of my patients' problems, safely and naturally. This path had already benefited so many of my patients that I felt a moral obligation to press ahead. After all, helping people obtain and maintain health and wellness naturally is what being a doctor should be all about.

Monica understood this simple principle. Because of her organizational abilities and deep convictions about serving our guests, she is now the executive vice president of our three enterprises and provides leadership for our ninety team members. Monica had challenged me to break away from the herd. How grateful I am to her for this counsel.

A TURNING POINT IN OUR HISTORY

The decision to be independent of any insurance arrangements was a pivotal moment in the evolution of the Hotze Health & Wellness Center. In choosing to work on our patients' behalf rather than on behalf of the insurance companies, we made a conscious choice to treat each person as a welcomed guest in our office rather than as a name in an appointment book or a five-minute slot in a hectic schedule.

This seemingly simple decision freed us to provide safe, effective, natural medical care and extraordinary hospitality and service to our guests. That's right, guests. We use this term because it helps us focus our thoughts on service and hospitality. We have modeled ourselves after fine hotels. The goal of the Hotze Health & Wellness Center is to enable our guests to enjoy a better quality of life. This commitment to improving the quality of life of our guests begins the very first time they call our office.

Twenty-five percent of our guests come from out of state. Why would so many people travel to the Hotze Health & Wellness Center if they were having their needs met back in their home states? Most of these individuals seek our help because they are at the end of their ropes. They have already seen numerous other physicians. They have been poked, prodded, and labeled. They have been treated like cattle or, worse, like an imposition on the medical staff and doctor. Many have been made to feel like hypochondriacs. They have been given prescription drugs, usually antidepressants, but they have not been given the things they need the most.

A person who is not feeling well has three basic needs: (1) to be listened to and understood, (2) to be cared for, and (3) to be appreciated. The medical treatment that is offered is really secondary to meeting these basic needs.

Every member of our staff is trained to understand these three basic needs. Each one knows the importance of listening intently, caring genuinely, and being grateful for the opportunity to serve our guests. Staff members are trained to anticipate our guests' needs and to exceed their expectations. When a guest walks into our center, she is the most important person to us, and she is treated as such by each staff member who assists her.

Occasionally some patients, usually women, feel uncomfortable being treated as guests. These individuals are used to making sacrifices for their spouses and children to ensure that their needs are met, but when it comes to fulfilling their own needs, they have difficulty asking for help. They find it unsettling to receive genuine care and concern because they have become so accustomed to long waits, discourteous staff, and little time or attention from their doctors. It's hard to imagine such negative environments fostering wellness.

If any retail business treated its customers the way that most doctors' offices treat their patients, then they would quickly be out of business. Physicians are able to get away with offering poor customer service because the masses view the medical profession with an almost religious sense of awe, fear, or respect.

MODERN MEDICINE IS THE NEW RELIGION

Webster's defines religion as "a cause, principle, or system of beliefs held to with ardor or faith." By this definition, modern medicine has all the trappings of a religion. This observation was first made by Robert Mendelsohn, M.D., in his book, *Confessions of a Medical Heretic*, which should be required reading for every first-year medical student.

The major medical centers are the cathedrals of this religious system, and the medical schools are the seminaries where novices are trained in the mysteries of medical doctrine and taught their priestly duties. At graduation, amid great pomp and circumstance, the title of doctor is conferred upon these thoroughly indoctrinated "clergy" members.

Filled with missionary zeal, the newly ordained minister dons the white coat and stethoscope that serve as the props of his priestly role and returns to the community to spread the gospel of health through drugs. He establishes his office as his chapel, and waits for the true believer, the suffering patient, to seek his care. He does not have to wait long.

When a patient arrives, she is escorted to the examination room, which is modern medicine's version of the confessional, where she waits nervously for the physician to appear. He makes his grand entrance, bearing the chart where he will note her complaints, take down her history, and enter his judgment as to her condition. After being asked what has brought her here, the patient describes her problem. She is then questioned and made to confess whether or not she drinks too much coffee or alcohol, eats too much junk food, smokes, worries too much, or fails to exercise.

When blood tests return within the normal range, the physician suggests that she has brought her health problems upon herself and offers her a drug solution to her problem. This is usually an antidepressant, which serves as the holy communion of the modern medical religion. To refuse to take this drug, or to ask whether there is any harm in it, is considered sacrilegious.

If you have difficulty understanding the religious nature of the medical profession, then the next time your physician prescribes a medication, a laboratory test, a diagnostic procedure, or a surgical operation, just ask him, "Why is this necessary?" If you persist in your questioning, then the physician will eventually say, "Trust me." Trusting without questioning is the basis of religious faith.

When medicine takes on religious overtones and its practices are considered sacred, patients are the primary victims. However, physicians who dare to challenge the ruling dogma may also be victimized by the medical establishment. That is what happened to a nineteenth-century Hungarian physician named Ignaz Semmelweis.

A MEDICAL HERETIC: VILIFIED, THEN VINDICATED

In the early 1800s, obstetrics was becoming a popular specialty among physicians because the invention of forceps had transformed childbirth into a surgical procedure. When physicians entered the domain of midwives, it proved disastrous for pregnant women. Tens of thousands of women suffered horrible, painful deaths from puerperal sepsis, also known as childbed fever, as a direct result of physician-assisted, hospital-based deliveries.

We now know that childbed fever is caused by a bacterial infection that develops in the vagina and spreads through the bloodstream to the entire body. However, before the germ theory was formulated in the late nineteenth century, physicians had no concept of bacterial infection. Some physicians blamed the disease on an imbalance of the blood humors in a woman's body, while others attributed it to miasma, a noxious atmosphere that was suspected of poisoning the air. Defects in a woman's constitution, the harmful effects of tight petticoats, solar or cosmic influences, and other theories were also advanced by various physicians and scientists.

The one point upon which nearly all physicians agreed was that childbed fever was unpreventable. They also knew that their usual treatments of bloodletting, purging, sweating, and fasting were ineffective in treating the disease. If anything, these procedures hastened the deaths of the unfortunate victims.

Ignaz Semmelweis (1818–1865) was just twenty-eight years old when he began a two-year assistantship in obstetrics in the First Obstetrical Clinic of the renowned Vienna General Hospital in Austria. Despite its reputation as one of the leading institutions of Europe, the Vienna General Hospital was experiencing periodic epidemics of childbed fever. During the mid-1800s, the mortality rate from childbed fever averaged 7–8 percent in the First Obstetrical Clinic, where deliveries were attended by physicians and medical students. In 1847, the year that Dr. Semmelweis began his assistantship, the mortality rate was almost 13 percent, meaning that one of every seven women who gave birth died of childbed fever.

Dr. Semmelweis was appalled by the suffering and deaths he witnessed on the wards. As a scientist who had spent several years studying pathology, he was convinced that the prevailing theories were wrong. He was determined to identify the cause of childbed fever and spent hundreds of hours performing autopsies, reading medical journals, poring over hospital records, and attempting to discover a pattern that would explain the cause of childbed fever.

Semmelweis found such a pattern when he examined the hospital's records and noted that the mortality rate from childbed fever in the First Obstetrical Clinic, where physicians and medical students attended deliveries, was six times higher than it was in the Second Obstetrical Clinic, where midwives performed deliveries. He was surprised to find that, outside of the hospital, the mortality rate from childbed fever was very low, even among poor women who gave birth in the streets and alleys of Vienna.

Semmelweis made an additional, very significant discovery when he observed that physicians and medical students often performed autopsies between deliveries and routinely went straight from the autopsy room to the delivery suite without washing their hands. Midwives, on the other hand, did not perform autopsies.

The final piece of the puzzle was revealed when a colleague of Semmelweis accidentally punctured his finger with a knife during an autopsy, developed an infection, and died. The autopsy revealed that this physician had died of a disease remarkably similar to childbed fever. Semmelweis recognized this resemblance and concluded that some unknown "cadaveric material" was responsible for his friend's fatal infection and also for childbed fever. He concluded that this unknown material was being transferred from the physician's hands to the patients during examinations and during delivery.

In order to prevent the spread of this disease from cadavers to patients, Dr. Semmelweis instituted a policy of hand washing between autopsies and the examination and delivery of women in labor. As a result, the mortality rate in the First Obstetrical Clinic dropped to approximately 2 percent, a level comparable to that seen in the midwives' clinic.

This led to an enormous controversy. Instead of embracing Semmelweis's theory, his colleagues vehemently opposed it. These physicians felt that their profession was divinely ordained. The notion that their own hands could be the instrument of disease was simply unacceptable to them. Instead, these physicians continued to hold to their belief that childbed fever was caused by an imbalance of blood humors or miasma.

Dr. Johann Klein, the chief of obstetrics at the hospital and Semmelweis's immediate superior, was outraged by Semmelweis's theory and by the newly instituted policy of hand washing that had been implemented. Despite the fact that there had been a dramatic reduction in the mortality rate from childbed fever, Klein refused to renew Semmelweis's assistantship. Semmelweis was ostracized by the medical establishment in Austria and fled to Hungary in disgrace.

Despite the resistance he had encountered in Vienna, Semmelweis remained committed to saving women's lives. He instituted a protocol of hand and instrument washing at the Hungarian hospital where he worked from 1851 to 1857. Although he managed to reduce the mortality rate from childbed fever to less than 1 percent on the maternity ward of this hospital, the physicians of Vienna remained hostile to his theory. It was not until almost half a century later that Semmelweis was posthumously vindicated and sterile techniques were widely instituted in hospitals in Western countries. Had Semmelweis's findings been accepted by the physicians of his time, tens of thousands of young mothers would have been spared death from childbed fever.

Dr. Semmelweis's vilification by his colleagues is not simply a curious anecdote in the annals of medicine. Throughout history, physicians who have challenged the dogmatic beliefs and dangerous practices of their colleagues have been branded as heretics, thrown into jail, or stripped of their medical licenses. Like Semmelweis, many physicians have died in disgrace, only to be vindicated later.

Hysteria, Hypochondria . . . or Hormonal Imbalance?

When the medical profession clings to outmoded theories and practices, it is the patients, usually women, who become the sacrificial lambs. Women have been victimized more frequently than men because the medical profession historically has been dominated by males and has always assumed a low view of women and their health problems.

For example, from the time of the ancient Greeks up to the early twentieth century, women whose emotions were judged as excessive were labeled as hysterics. Hippocrates believed that hysteria was caused by the movement of the uterus from its normal position in the pelvis to other parts of the body. The term hysteria is derived from the Greek word "hyster," which means uterus. Hysteria literally means "wandering uterus." In other historical periods, hysteria has been attributed to demonic possession, sexual repression, or an attention-seeking personality.

A more likely explanation for the symptoms of women labeled as hysterics is female hormonal imbalance, which can be remedied easily with bioidentical hormone replacement. However, the female hormones were not even discovered until the 1930s. So for two thousand years, women whose emotions were judged to be excessive were confined in insane asylums or subjected to barbaric treatment such as binding, fasting, or purging. Some were even burned at the stake as witches.

In the more "modern" era of the twentieth century, women with symptoms of hysteria have been given electrical shock therapy or subjected to so many medical and surgical interventions that the disease was given a new name: "thick file syndrome." Innumerable times during my medical career I have heard other physicians refer to these women as "crocks."

Today, women are more likely to be labeled hypochondriacs than hysterics, but the implication that women are lesser creatures persists. Women whose blood tests are "normal" but who insist that they do not feel well are viewed as emotionally unstable and mentally disturbed. As I mentioned in an earlier chapter, during medical school I was taught by one of my professors that any woman in midlife who had more than one major complaint should be considered a hypochondriac and prescribed an antidepressant. This explains why the overwhelming majority of antidepressant prescriptions are given to women between the ages of thirty-five and fifty-five.

If women are inordinately labeled as neurotic or crazy, they are also inordinately exposed to unnecessary surgery. In *Confessions of a Medical Heretic*, Dr. Mendelsohn reported that 43 percent of hysterectomies performed at six New York hospitals were later judged medically unnecessary. When Dr. Mendelsohn's book was published in 1979, approximately 750,000 women underwent hysterectomies each year, which means that roughly 300,000 women were needlessly castrated in one year.

In 1988, gynecologist Vicki Hufnagel, M.D., wrote a book called *No More Hysterectomies* that exposed how little this situation had improved. According to her research, the number of hysterectomies performed had declined annually during the intervening decade, but the number of hysterectomies that were medically unnecessary had skyrocketed. By her estimation, up to 90 percent of all hysterectomies could have been avoided, had other options been explored and offered to women.

But the tragedy doesn't end with this statistic. Millions of women who underwent surgical menopause at the urging of their physician, and millions more who passed through menopause with their uteruses intact, have been prescribed counterfeit hormones such as Premarin and Provera to ease their hot flashes, protect their bones, and reduce their risk of heart disease. However, not only did these drugs fail to reduce their risk of heart disease, they actually increased risk. As I reported in chapter 7, the Women's Health Initiative (WHI) was halted three years early because women using counterfeit hormones had an increased risk of breast cancer, heart disease, stroke, and pulmonary embolism compared to women who were given a placebo.

Despite the numerous negative reports from the WHI, the Million Women Study, and other studies, the counterfeit hormones have not gone away. The drug companies will not voluntarily give up on such a profitable pharmaceutical product. Wyeth's solution to the bad press about their product, Prempro, has been to begin promoting a new low-dose Prempro, which I call "Prempro Lite."

DON'T GET CAUGHT IN A STAMPEDE

Pharmaceutical companies, like life insurance companies, are publicly traded businesses listed on the stock exchanges. Their primary purpose is to make a profit. While this may be good for the stockholders, it is not always in the best interest of patients. These companies are solely interested in promoting the use of drugs to address health problems, despite the fact that drugs only treat the symptoms of illness and never address the underlying cause. Drugs are unnatural chemicals that have been made in pharmaceutical laboratories, and their use is usually accompanied by a host of adverse side effects. Remember that drugs must be detoxified by your body, and as you get older your body is less able to eliminate drug toxins.

As I have explained in the preceding chapters, illness is not caused by a lack of prescription drugs. Most illnesses are due to poor dietary habits and nutrition, lack of exercise, allergic disorders that weaken the immune system and make it more prone to infection, yeast overgrowth due to overuse of antibiotics, an imbalance and decline in the body's production of thyroid and sex hormones, and stressed adrenal glands. All of these factors can be addressed safely, effectively, and naturally without drugs.

Physicians who obtain their continuing education at conferences sponsored by the drug companies are unaware of this, because they are indoctrinated with the dogma being promoted by these drug companies. Physicians are often too willing to believe whatever the drug companies tell them about a product's safety and effectiveness.

A recent example of this is the Vioxx debacle. Vioxx is a member of a new class of painkillers called COX-2 inhibitors used to treat arthritis. Vioxx received a speedy approval from the FDA in 1999, but it was pulled from the market in October, 2004 after it was shown to dramatically increase the risk of heart attacks in those who used it. Merck, the maker of Vioxx, had been warned by researchers of this potential problem in 1998. Despite this, Merck released and promoted Vioxx to overly trusting physicians and to the public.

Furthermore, physicians who are enrolled in health maintenance organizations have their hands tied. They must treat you using drugs, and specifically the drugs that the HMO has approved, rather than with safer, natural therapies.

People who get caught in stampedes get trampled. To protect your health you simply must get out of HMOs and hire a doctor who will work for you rather than for the insurance companies or for the government. You are in a better position than any insurance clerk or government bureaucrat to choose the type of medical care you should seek.

Following the herd will never lead you to optimal health or success in life. You can take the first courageous step toward obtaining and maintaining health and wellness naturally by breaking out of the herd, taking charge of your health, and sidestepping the stampede toward drugs.

CHAPTER 13

Get Your Life Back!

This book opened with the story of Maggie, whose treatment by the physicians she consulted clearly demonstrates the problem with modern medicine. Instead of being listened to, cared for, and appreciated, Maggie was made to feel like she was an imposition on the medical staff and doctors. When she failed to get well in this "mismanaged care" environment, she was labeled a hypochondriac.

Fortunately, Maggie recognized that something was not right with her body, even though the doctors she had consulted told her that her blood tests were perfectly normal. Because of her determination to get to the root cause of her problems, she took charge of her health and did what was necessary to get her life back.

Maggie's story is not unique. My staff and I have seen thousands of our guests get their lives back by following the comprehensive program outlined in this book. Because we have witnessed firsthand the dramatic improvement in health and wellness that can be obtained with the proper use of natural, bioidentical hormones, we believe it is our moral imperative to bring information about this program to a wider audience.

We are leading a Wellness Revolution that advances a new model of health care for our society. Unlike the prevailing medical model, which uses drugs and surgery to treat illness or manage symptoms, this new model is built around a regimen of biologically identical hormones, Armour Thyroid, and other natural treatments to help individuals obtain and maintain health and wellness.

This Wellness Revolution, like all revolutions, will not be embraced by the vested interests in society. The medical establishment, the pharmaceutical companies, the FDA, and the insurance industry will be throwing up roadblocks and opposition every step of the way. These groups are profiting handsomely from the status quo and have no desire to promote changes in health care that benefit patients but decrease profits.

Fortunately, there is already a cadre of physicians around the country who understand the need for change and who have embraced the concepts of the Wellness Revolution. Many more are being trained by the American Academy of Biologically Identical Hormone Therapy (AABIHT), which I established in 2003. The use of bioidentical hormones is not taught in medical schools, and the drug companies are definitely not going to promote this alternative to their drug therapy. This is why the AABIHT was established. The goals of this academy are to standardize the use of bioidentical hormone therapy and to ensure that properly trained physicians can bring this therapy to the women and men of this country.

Thousands of women and men have joined the Wellness Revolution, simply by refusing to settle for second-class treatment by their physicians. These individuals have taken charge of their health and have done what is necessary to get their lives back. Maggie and the other guests of the Hotze Health & Wellness Center whose stories I have shared in this book, and the thousands others whose stories were not included, are the true medical heroes and heroines.

If you are sick and tired of being sick and tired, then I hope that these stories have inspired you to take charge of your own health and get your life back. Nobody will care more about your health than you will. You simply cannot wait for conventional, mainstream physicians to realize that the "disease and drug" model of medicine is as ill conceived as was the medieval notion that the world is flat.

If you have been told by your physician that you will just have to learn to live with your health problems, then allow me to recommend that you consider changing doctors. Find a physician who will listen to you with understanding, care deeply about your health and well-being, and serve you with compassion and respect. Find a physician whose staff members are dedicated to providing you with the finest personal attention and medical care. Find a physician who is trained in the use of natural, bioidentical hormones and who is committed to helping you obtain and maintain health and wellness naturally so that you may enjoy a better quality of life. Find a physician who will guide you onto a lifelong path of health and wellness.

After having been on our program, the most common comment our guests make to us is this: "Thank you for giving me my life back." This is my desire for you, too, that you get your life back. If you will write this down as your goal and follow the pathway to health and wellness that I have outlined in this book, then I am convinced that you will be successful.

Appendix A
Health Questionnaires

Test Yourself for Allergies

Do you have allergies? This questionnaire is similar to the one we give to guests at the Hotze Health & Wellness Center to help determine whether or not they are suffering from allergies. Read each question carefully, and record the number next to the question if it applies to you. When you finish, add up the numbers you have recorded and make note of your total score.

Do you experience fatigue?	3
Do you have frequent headaches?	2
Do you experience sneezing, postnasal drainage, or itching of the nose?	4
Do you have frequent colds?	2
Do you experience dizziness?	4
Do you get sinus infections every year?	3
Do your eyes itch, water, get red, or swell?	4

Do you have recurrent ear infections?   2

Do you have asthma, wheezing, tightness
in the chest, or chronic cough?   4

Do you have skin problems such as eczema,
skin rashes, itching, or hives?   3

Do you have indigestion, bloating,
diarrhea, or constipation?   1

Do your symptoms worsen during a
particular season, such as the spring or fall?   4

Do your symptoms change when you go
indoors or outdoors?   3

Are your symptoms worse in parks or grassy areas?   4

Are your symptoms worse in the bedroom after
going to bed, or in the morning upon arising?   2

Do you awaken in the middle of the night
with congestion?   2

Are your symptoms worse when you come
into contact with dust?   4

Are your symptoms worse around animals?   2

Do you have any blood relatives with allergies?   2

Do you have mood swings or feel depressed
for no reason?   1

Do you have recurrent yeast infections, jock itch,
athlete's foot, or fungus under your toenails?   2

Do you develop symptoms after eating or
drinking certain foods?   2

Do you sometimes feel stimulated, hyperactive,
or fatigued after meals?   2

Do you have dark circles under your eyes?   2

Do you have a crease across the bridge of your nose?   2

TOTAL SCORE

If your total score is less than 9, it is not likely that you have allergies. A score between 9 and 12 suggests the possibility of allergies. A score between 13 and 30 means that allergies are probable, while a score above 30 indicates that allergies are very likely.

TEST YOURSELF FOR YEAST OVERGROWTH

Do you have yeast overgrowth (candidiasis)? This questionnaire is similar to the one we give to guests at the Hotze Health & Wellness Center to help determine whether or not they are suffering from yeast overgrowth. Read each question carefully, and record the number next to the question if it applies to you. When you finish, add up the numbers you have recorded and make note of your total score.

Do you experience fatigue?   3

Do you feel lethargic?   2

Do you have recurrent vaginal yeast infections?   4

Have you taken antibiotics multiple times
during your life?   3

Do you have abdominal bloating, cramping, or gas?   3

Do you have indigestion or heartburn?   2

Do you have abnormal bodily reactions to
wine, beer, or liquor, such as flushing, headache,
sinus congestion, or itchy skin?   2

Do you crave sugar or bread products?   2

Do you have difficulty concentrating?   1

Do you have depressed moods?	1
Do you develop skin rashes or hives?	2
Do you have athlete's foot?	4
Do you have jock itch?	4
Do you experience rectal itching?	3
Do you have fungal infections under your toenails or fingernails?	3
Do you have allergy symptoms?	1
Do you have recurrent respiratory infections?	1
Do you experience joint pain?	1
Do you experience muscle pain?	1

TOTAL SCORE

If your total score is less than 10, it is not likely that you have yeast overgrowth. A score between 10 and 16 suggests that yeast overgrowth is a possibility. A score above 16 indicates that yeast overgrowth is very likely.

Test Yourself for Low Thyroid Function

Do you have low thyroid function (hypothyroidism)? This questionnaire is similar to the one we give to guests at the Hotze Health & Wellness Center to help determine whether or not they are suffering from low thyroid function. Read each question carefully, and record the number next to the question if it applies to you. When you finish, add up the numbers you have recorded and make note of your total score.

Do you experience fatigue?	4
Do you have elevated cholesterol?	4
Do you have difficulty losing weight?	2
Do you have cold hands and feet?	2
Are you sensitive to cold?	2
Do you have difficulty thinking?	2
Do you find it hard to concentrate?	2
Do you have poor short-term memory?	2
Are your moods depressed?	2
Are you experiencing hair loss?	2

Do you have fewer than one bowel movement a day?   2

Do you have dry skin?   2

Do you have itchy skin during the winter?   1

Do you experience fluid retention?   2

Do you have recurrent headaches?   1

Do you sleep restlessly?   1

Are you tired when you awaken?   2

Do you have afternoon fatigue?   2

Do you experience tingling or numbness
in your hands or feet?   2

Do you experience decreased sweating?   2

Have you had problems with infertility
or miscarriages?   2

Do you have recurrent infections?   2

Do your muscles ache?   2

Do you have joint pain?   2

Do you have thinning of your eyebrows or eyelashes?   2

Is your tongue enlarged with teeth indentations?	2
Is your skin pasty, puffy, or pale?	2
Do you have decreased body hair?	2
Is your voice hoarse?	1
Do you have a slow pulse?	2
Do you have low blood pressure?	2
Does your body temperature run below the normal 98.6 ?	4
Do you have sleep apnea?	2

TOTAL SCORE

If your total score is less than 11, it is not likely that you have low thyroid function. A score between 11 and 30 suggests that low thyroid function is a possibility. A score above 30 indicates that low thyroid function is very likely.

Test Yourself for Estrogen Dominance

Do you have estrogen dominance (progesterone deficiency)? This questionnaire is similar to the one we give to women at the Hotze Health & Wellness Center to help determine whether or not they are suffering from estrogen dominance. Read each question carefully, and record the number next to the question if it applies to you. When you finish, add up the numbers you have recorded and make note of your total score.

Do you experience premenstrual breast tenderness?	4
Do you have premenstrual mood swings?	4
Do you experience premenstrual fluid retention and weight gain?	4
Do you experience premenstrual headaches?	4
Do you experience migraine headaches?	3
Do you experience severe menstrual cramps?	4
Do you have heavy periods with clotting?	3
Do you have irregular menstrual cycles?	3
Do you have uterine fibroids?	3
Do you have fibrocystic breast disease?	3

Do you have endometriosis?	2
Have you had problems with infertility?	2
Have you had more than one miscarriage?	2
Do you experience joint pain?	1
Do you experience muscle pain?	1
Do you have a decreased libido?	3
Do you have anxiety or panic attacks?	2

TOTAL SCORE

If your total score is less than 5, it is not likely that you have estrogen dominance. A score between 5 and 8 suggests the possibility of estrogen dominance. A score between 9 and 20 means that estrogen dominance is probable, while a score above 20 indicates that estrogen dominance is very likely.

Test Yourself for Low Estrogen Levels

Are you in perimenopause or menopause? This questionnaire is similar to the one we give to women at the Hotze Health & Wellness Center to help determine whether or not they are suffering from perimenopausal or menopausal symptoms of low estrogen. Read each question carefully, and record the number next to the question if it applies to you. When you finish, add up the numbers you have recorded and make note of your total score.

Do you have hot flashes?	4
Do you have night sweats?	4
Do you have vaginal dryness?	3
Do you urinate frequently?	2
Are you depressed?	2
Do you have difficulty sleeping?	3
Have you lost interest in sex?	2
Have your periods ceased?	4

TOTAL SCORE

If your total score is less than 5, it is not likely that you have low estrogen. A score between 5 and 9 suggests that low estrogen is a possibility. A score above 9 indicates that low estrogen is very likely.

TEST YOURSELF FOR LOW TESTOSTERONE LEVELS (FOR MEN)

Do you have low testosterone levels? This questionnaire is similar to the one we give to men at the Hotze Health & Wellness Center to help determine whether or not they are suffering from low testosterone levels. Read each question carefully, and record the number next to the question if it applies to you. When you finish, add up the numbers you have recorded and make note of your total score.

Do you experience fatigue?	2
Do you feel a lack of drive?	3
Do you lack initiative?	3
Are you less assertive?	3
Do you have a decline in your sense of well-being?	2
Do you have depressed moods?	2
Are you frequently irritable?	2
Has your self-confidence declined?	2
Do you find it difficult to set goals?	2
Do you have a difficult time making decisions?	2

Have you had a decline in your mental sharpness?   2

Has your stamina and endurance lessened?   2

Have you lost muscle mass, strength, or tone?   4

Have you gained body fat around your waist?   2

Do you have elevated cholesterol?   2

Has your libido decreased?   4

Has your sexual ability declined?   2

Is it difficult to obtain or maintain an erection?   2

Do you have sleep apnea?   2

TOTAL SCORE

If your total score is less than 7, it is not likely that you have low testosterone. A score between 7 and 20 suggests that low testosterone is a possibility. A score above 20 indicates that low testosterone is very likely.

TEST YOURSELF FOR ADRENAL FATIGUE

Do you have adrenal fatigue? This questionnaire is similar to the one we give to guests at the Hotze Health & Wellness Center to help determine whether or not they are suffering from adrenal fatigue. Read each question carefully, and record the number next to the question if it applies to you. When you finish, add up the numbers you have recorded and make note of your total score.

Do you experience fatigue? 3

Do you have allergies? 3

Do you have asthma? 3

Do you have recurrent infections? 3

Are you under severe emotional stress? 3

Do you suffer from chronic pain or physical stress? 3

Do you have low blood pressure? 2

Do you have a low pulse rate (fewer than 70 beats per minute with no exercise)? 2

When you rise quickly, do you feel as though you might pass out? 2

Do you experience depressed moods?	2
Do you experience joint pain?	2
Do you have muscle pain?	2
Do you have low libido?	2
Do you have hair loss?	2
Do you have anxiety attacks?	2

TOTAL SCORE

If your total score is less than 7, it is not likely that you have adrenal fatigue. A score between 7 and 12 suggests that adrenal fatigue is a possibility. A score above 12 indicates that adrenal fatigue is very likely.

Appendix B
More on Nutrition

In chapter 10, I wrote a simple synopsis of the healthy eating program that I recommend to my patients. This eating program balances protein, vegetables and fruits while minimizing starchy carbohydrates.

Numerous books have been written on this subject, such as *Sugar Busters*, *The Atkins Diet*, and *The Zone: A Dietary Road Map to Lose Weight Permanently* to name a few.

In this appendix, I will explain why this eating program works.

A Tale of Two Hormones

I've been talking quite a bit about hormones in this book, because hormones are key regulators of virtually every metabolic process in your body. Many of these hormones operate in pairs, with the effects of one hormone offsetting the effects of another. You may recall from my discussion of the female hormones that estrogen and progesterone have different, often opposing actions. The optimal balance of these two hormones is crucial to a woman's health and well-being.

The same holds true for two hormones produced by the pancreas: insulin and glucagon. Insulin's primary role is to "push" glucose out of the blood and into the cells, where it is either used for energy or stored as glycogen or fat. The hormone glucagon has exactly the opposite effect: it "pulls" glucose out of the liver and into the bloodstream.

The ebb and flow of insulin and glucagon alternate throughout the day. Each time you eat a meal, insulin is secreted by the pancreas. Like a courier delivering a time-sensitive package, insulin "knocks" on the door of the cell, then ushers glucose out of the bloodstream and into the cell. In the fasting state—for example, when you first wake up in the morning—this pathway is reversed: your pancreas secretes glucagon, which promotes the conversion of stored carbohydrates or fat to sugar, followed by its release into the bloodstream.

Several things can go wrong with this hormonal dance. If the insulin-secreting beta cells of the pancreas are damaged or destroyed, then the body will produce too little insulin. The result is type 1 or insulin-dependent diabetes, a serious metabolic disorder that causes blood glucose levels to soar dangerously high. This in turn causes excessive urination, the body's attempt to rid itself of glucose; excessive thirst, to replace the water lost through urination; ravenous hunger, due to the malnourishment of cells; and weight loss, a consequence of the inability of the body to take in glucose. Unless insulin is provided from outside the body, the individual with type 1 diabetes will literally waste away from malnutrition.

Only 10 percent of diabetics have type 1 diabetes. The remaining 90 percent suffer from type 2 diabetes. Before 1980, this condition was called adult-onset diabetes, reflecting its status as a disease primarily affecting those over the age of forty. Unfortunately, "adult onset" no longer holds true. Thanks to the American love affair with refined carbohydrates and the increase in childhood obesity, even teenagers are being diagnosed with this disease, and it is now referred to as either type 2 diabetes or non-insulin-dependent diabetes.

As its name suggests, non-insulin-dependent diabetes is not caused by inadequate production of insulin. Instead, it is characterized by an inability of the body to use insulin effectively. In other words, the problem is not a lack of insulin but a decline in the sensitivity of cells to the signals of this messenger hormone, a condition called insulin resistance. Even though there is plenty of insulin in circulation, the effect of insulin resistance is the same as that of insulin insufficiency: glucose cannot get into cells, and as a result, blood sugar levels remain elevated.

While all type 2 diabetics have insulin resistance, not all individuals with insulin resistance have type 2 diabetes. In fact, almost one-third of Americans suffer from insulin resistance, but only 5–10 percent of these individuals eventually develop type 2 diabetes. The remaining 90–95 percent may not suffer the ill effects of high blood glucose levels, but they have an equally serious problem: hyperinsulinemia, or chronically elevated levels of insulin in the blood.

The Hazards of High Insulin Levels—Syndrome X

At first glance, hyperinsulinemia sounds like a clever solution to the problem of insulin resistance. After all, if the cells cannot "hear" the message of insulin, doesn't it make sense to make the message louder? This is exactly what the pancreas does. Whereas a healthy individual produces about 31 units of insulin a day, the individual with insulin resistance may produce over 100 units—three times as much—in order to "push" glucose out of the blood and into the cells.

Hyperinsulinemia prevents blood glucose levels from remaining chronically elevated, at least in the early stages, before the onset of full-blown type 2 diabetes. However, the body's attempt to compensate for insulin resistance by increasing insulin production creates many new problems. Here are just a few of the well-documented effects of hyperinsulinemia:

- Too much insulin promotes salt retention, which contributes to high blood pressure. Half of all patients with hypertension have insulin resistance and hyperinsulinemia.
- Too much insulin wreaks havoc on cholesterol levels. It causes triglyceride levels to go up, while levels of beneficial HDL cholesterol go down. It also promotes the formation of smaller, more dangerous LDL particles.
- Too much insulin promotes the synthesis of inflammatory chemicals that damage the inner lining of the arteries, making it easier for cholesterol-rich plaques to adhere.
- Too much insulin increases the concentration of uric acid in the blood, which can lead to the development of gouty arthritis. An elevated level of uric acid, a waste product excreted through the kidneys, is also an independent risk factor for heart disease and stroke.
- Too much insulin promotes weight gain, especially in the abdominal area.

This pattern of elevated insulin levels, high blood pressure, high triglycerides, low HDL, increased inflammation, elevated uric acid, and abdominal obesity is seen so frequently in physicians' offices that it even has a name, Syndrome X. Gerald

Reaven, M.D., first described this pattern in 1988 at the annual meeting of the American Diabetes Association. Since then, researchers have been studying the causes and consequences of Syndrome X in earnest. We now know that individuals who fit this profile have a significantly higher risk of heart disease. We also know that hyperinsulinemia is the defining feature of Syndrome X and the underlying cause of much of the damage to the heart, blood vessels, kidneys, and other vital organs.

The moral of the story? Do everything you can to keep insulin levels in the low normal range. Here's how.

Curb Your Sweet Tooth

If keeping insulin levels in the low normal range is the key to optimal health and well-being, then eating the right types and amounts of carbohydrates is the key to regulating insulin levels. The body converts all carbohydrates to glucose, which is released into the bloodstream, prompting the pancreas to secrete insulin. But not all carbohydrates are equal in this regard. How quickly a carbohydrate-rich food enters the bloodstream is governed primarily by three factors: the structure of its sugars, its fiber content, and the amount of fat it contains.

GLUCOSE   FRUCTOSE   GALACTOSE

Figure 15. The monosaccharides.

The three monosaccharides have the same chemical formula but different chemical structures. Glucose, also called blood sugar or dextrose, is the body's primary energy source. Fructose, found in fruit and honey, is the sweetest of the simple sugars. Galactose is a building block of the disaccharide lactose (milk sugar).

The simplest of the simple sugars are the monosaccharides glucose, fructose, and galactose. The disaccharides—sucrose, maltose, and lactose—have a slightly more complicated structure, consisting of one molecule of glucose plus a second molecule of glucose, fructose, or galactose. All six of these sugars are classified as simple carbohydrates, and all are rapidly absorbed by the liver. However, only glucose can be released directly into the bloodstream. The other simple carbohydrates must first be broken down into individual molecules of glucose.

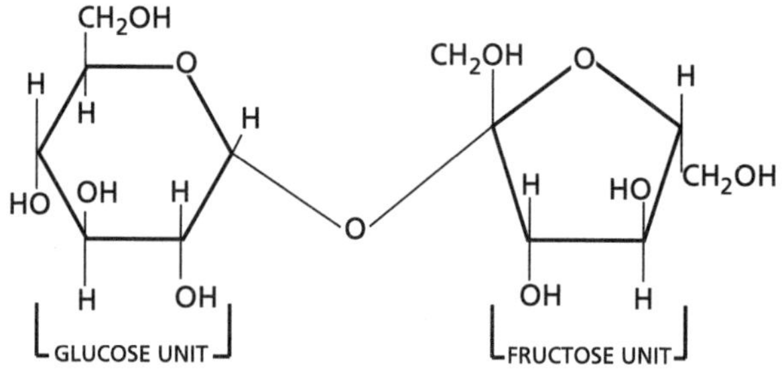

Figure 16. The disaccharide sucrose.
A disaccharide (di = two) is formed when one molecule of glucose is combined with a second molecule of glucose, fructose, or galactose. For example, the disaccharide sucrose (table sugar) is formed from glucose plus fructose.

Though starches are classified as complex carbohydrates, their structure is simply a series of glucose molecules linked together, and the bonds between these glucose molecules are easily broken. For this reason, starches act much like simple sugars in the body. They are rapidly absorbed by the liver and are released fairly quickly into the bloodstream.

Only fiber truly deserves to be called a complex carbohydrate because only fiber has a structure that cannot be broken down by digestive enzymes. Fiber is not absorbed by the body, and it does not raise insulin levels. Even more important for keeping insulin levels low, fiber delays the release of glucose into the bloodstream. This is one reason why fiber-rich whole fruits have a less dramatic effect on blood sugar levels than fruit juices, especially pulpless juices.

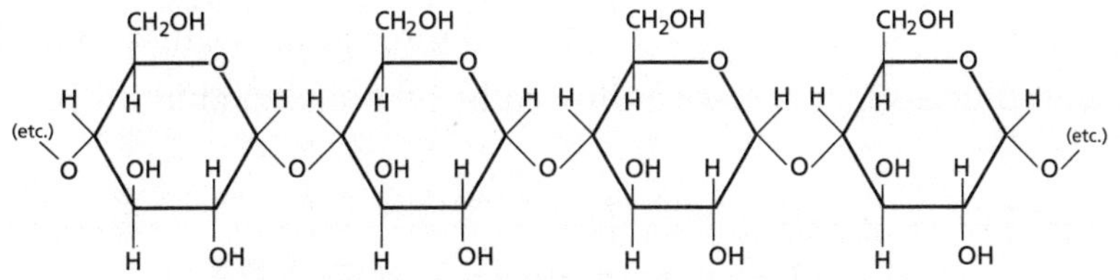

Figure 17. The starch amylose.

Like all starches, amylose is a polysaccharide (poly = many), a giant molecule composed of hundreds or thousands of glucose molecules linked together. Starches are easily broken down into individual glucose molecules by digestive enzymes, so they cause blood sugar to rise rapidly.

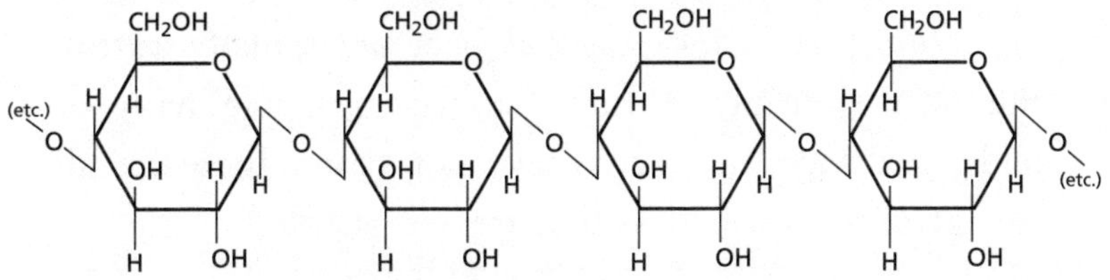

Figure 18. The fiber cellulose.

Like all fibers, cellulose is found only in plant foods — vegetables, fruits, grains, and legumes. Fibers cannot be broken down into individual monosaccharides by digestive enzymes, so they do not cause blood sugar to rise rapidly.

Fat also slows the release of glucose into the bloodstream. Though some carbohydrate-rich foods such as vegetables and fruits are virtually fat-free, you can help keep blood sugar levels steady by consuming a small amount of fat along with these foods.

While these three variables—the structure of the sugars, the fiber content, and the presence of fat—can interact in countless ways, scientists have found a simple method to quantify the effects of carbohydrate-containing foods on blood sugar levels. Called the glycemic index, it is a measure of the rate at which blood glucose levels rise two to three hours after you've eaten a food. Foods with a low glycemic index (most vegetables and fruits) cause a gradual rise in blood sugar levels, followed by a gradual decline. Insulin levels usually show a similarly graceful curve. On the other hand, foods with a high glycemic index (starchy vegetables, tropical fruits, and most grains) cause a rapid rise in blood sugar, usually followed by an equally rapid drop.

READ LABELS FOR HIDDEN SUGARS

Sugar can appear in many disguises and in foods that are not generally thought of as sweet, such as soups and salad dressings. Check labels for sucrose, dextrose, lactose, and other "-ose" words, as well as corn syrup and high-fructose corn syrup (HFCS), cane sugar, beet sugar, maltodextrin, fruit juice concentrate, honey, molasses, maple syrup or solids, and corn, rice, or barley malt syrup. These are all high-glycemic sweeteners that are best avoided.

Eating a lot of high-glycemic foods can tax your body's blood sugar mechanisms, zap you of energy, impair your thinking, and make you feel irritable or depressed. If optimal health and peak performance are your goals, then this is one roller coaster ride you do not want to take. It's also a bad idea if you're trying to lose weight, because insulin promotes the storage of fat. Even worse, the steep drop in blood sugar a few hours after a high-glycemic meal or snack makes you ravenously hungry. It's easy to overeat when your blood sugar has bottomed out.

Straight Facts About Fats

If carbohydrates have been wrongly characterized as health foods, then fats have been just as wrongly depicted as dietary villains. The fact is that fats are essential to life. Fats are required for the absorption of the fat-soluble vitamins (A, D, E, and K), they serve as essential components of cell membranes, and they are used to make hormones. Fats insulate our bodies, cushion and protect our organs, and provide a concentrated source of energy. Dietary fats add flavor to foods, making them taste better, and slow the release of glucose into the bloodstream, helping to keep blood sugar levels steady.

However, just as some types of carbohydrates are more healthful than others, so are some fats. Most dietary fats consist of a mixture of three different types of fatty acids—saturated, monounsaturated, and polyunsaturated—but usually one of these types predominates. Most animal fats and tropical oils consist primarily of saturated fatty acids; olive and canola oil are primarily monounsaturated; and corn, safflower, sunflower, and other vegetable and seed oils are predominantly polyunsaturated. Each of these types of fatty acids has a different structure, different chemical properties, and different effects on your health.

The Skinny on Saturated Fatty Acids

There are two types of fatty acids: saturated fatty acids and unsaturated fatty acids. Saturated fatty acids are long, straight molecules consisting of a skeleton of carbon atoms, each of which is bonded to its neighboring carbon atoms and to two hydrogen atoms. Much like a commuter train in which every seat is filled, a fatty acid that is "saturated" has all of its carbon atoms occupied. For this reason, saturated fatty acids are not very chemically reactive, especially when compared to the mono- and polyunsaturated fatty acids. This lack of reactivity means that their role in your body is somewhat limited. Saturated fatty acids participate in building cell membranes and they are burned for fuel, but any excess saturated fatty acids beyond your body's needs are stored as body fat. Saturated fatty acids also lower your metabolism, making it harder for you to lose weight.

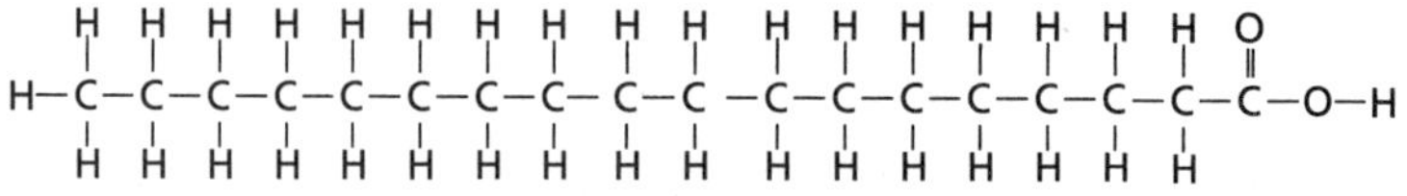

Figure 19. Stearic acid.
Stearic acid, found in beef, pork, butter, and cocoa butter, is called a saturated fatty acid because it contains only single bonds between its carbon atoms (the carbons are "saturated" with hydrogen).

Saturated fatty acids tend to clump together rather than dispersing through other fluids. This "clumping" activity can clog a kitchen drain, but it has even more serious implications for the health of your arteries. Saturated fatty acids cause blood platelets to stick together, impairing circulation, and they can be deposited in your artery walls, contributing to the formation of fatty streaks and plaques. In addition, excess saturated fats from meat, dairy products, and tropical oils are the major dietary contributor to LDL cholesterol levels. A diet high in saturated fats also contributes to insulin resistance, a prediabetic condition with a host of negative health consequences.

Because your body can produce all of the saturated fatty acids it needs, I recommend that you minimize your intake of foods that are high in saturated fat, such as lard, fatty cuts of meat, and dairy products.

THE BENEFITS OF DOUBLE BONDS

Unsaturated fatty acids differ from saturated fatty acids in that some of their carbon atoms are not bonded to hydrogen atoms but instead have formed a double bond with a neighboring carbon atom. The double bond is like a "reserved" sign on the seat of a train—it is a placeholder that can be used to form bonds with other molecules. A monounsaturated fatty acid has just one of these double bonds ("mono" means *one*), while a polyunsaturated fatty acid has two or more ("poly" means *many*). These double bonds make unsaturated fatty acids more chemically reactive than saturated fatty acids.

Figure 20. Oleic acid and linoleic acid.

Oleic acid, found in olive oil, is called a monounsaturated fatty acid because it contains one double bond between carbon atoms. Linoleic acid, found in many seed and vegetable oils, is called a polyunsaturated fatty acid because it contains more than one double bond between carbon atoms.

The double bonds in an unsaturated fatty acid have another effect on this molecule's properties: they create a kink in the carbon skeleton, giving the molecule a curved configuration that is quite different from the structure of a saturated fatty acid. This "kink in the chain" makes it difficult for unsaturated fatty acid molecules to clump together, which is good news for your kitchen drain and even better news for your arteries. In your bloodstream, these fats prevent blood platelets from clumping together and promote healthy circulation.

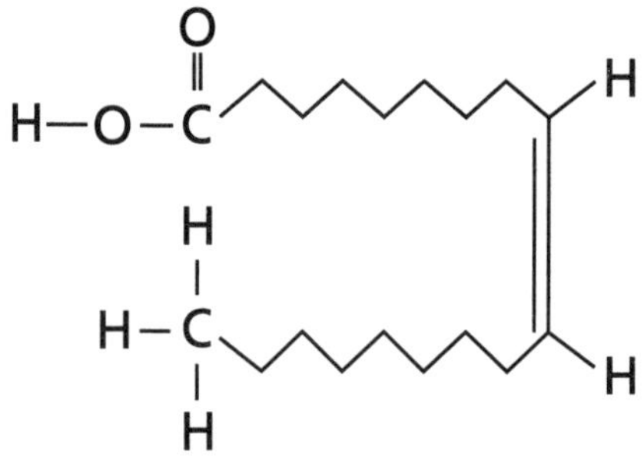

Figure 21. The cis configuration of oleic acid.
In nature, most unsaturated fatty acids exist in a U-shaped cis configuration. When oils containing unsaturated fatty acids are heated or partially hydrogenated, some of the cis fatty acids are transformed into unnatural and unhealthy trans fatty acids. (See Figure 21.)

Monounsaturated fatty acids, found abundantly in olives and olive oil, are a key component of the traditional Mediterranean diet, which is consumed by inhabitants of Spain, southern France, Italy, and Greece. A number of studies have found that populations adhering to a Mediterranean-type diet have reduced rates of obesity, cardiovascular disease, and cancer in comparison to those following a typical Western diet.

Monounsaturated fatty acids have several virtues. They don't raise LDL cholesterol levels and they don't affect insulin levels, but they do promote supple arteries. Though they are more chemically reactive than saturated fatty acids, they are less so than polyunsaturated fatty acids. This makes them more stable and less prone to oxidation when heated than polyunsaturated fatty acids, and it is why I recommend that you use a monounsaturated oil—olive oil or canola oil—when you cook or bake. I also recommend that you add almonds, macadamias, pistachios, pecans, hazelnuts, cashews, olives, and avocados to your diet. All of these foods are good sources of monounsaturated fatty acids.

A Delicate Balance

Because polyunsaturated fatty acids contain multiple double bonds, they are the most chemically reactive of the fatty acids and the ones that serve the most important and varied functions in your body. For example, although all three types of fats participate in forming cell membranes, polyunsaturated fatty acids are the ones that give a cell membrane its fluidity and enable it to act as a selective barrier. Cell membranes formed of lesser fats lack structural integrity, which can threaten the health of the entire cell.

Polyunsaturated fatty acids also serve as precursors to hormones called eicosanoids, which are key regulators of cellular function. Just as endocrine hormones often come in pairs with opposing functions, so too do many of the eicosanoids. Some cause your blood vessels to constrict, while others cause them to relax and widen. Some promote inflammation, while others have an anti-inflammatory effect. Some make the blood more viscous, while others enhance the fluidity of blood.

The optimal functioning of your cardiovascular system, immune system, and nervous system depends on having the right balance of eicosanoids, which in turn depends on having the right balance of fats in your diet. Minimizing your intake of animal fats and maximizing your intake of monounsaturated fats is the first step. The next step is to get the right balance of two polyunsaturated fatty acids, an omega-6 fatty acid called linoleic acid (LA) and an omega-3 fatty acid called alpha-linolenic acid (ALA).

LA and ALA are known as essential fatty acids because they are essential for good health, yet our bodies cannot manufacture them. The only way to get these essential fats is by eating foods that contain them or taking nutritional supplements. Most of us get plenty of LA from our diet, as this omega-6 fatty acid is abundant in the vegetable and seed oils used in many of the foods we eat. In contrast, there are few good food sources of the omega-3 fatty acid ALA. Soybeans and soybean oil contain some, as do walnuts and wheat germ. But the best source of ALA is flaxseed oil, which is hardly a staple food in this country. This is why I recommend that you take a flaxseed oil supplement. It's a simple way to help correct the imbalance of essential fats in your body.

Another option is to eat salmon, mackerel, trout, sardines, or other cold-water species of fish several times a week. Though the oil from these fish does not contain ALA, it contains a beneficial omega-3 fatty acid called eicosapentaenoic acid (EPA), which is a close relative of ALA. In fact, your body converts the ALA you consume to EPA, and then uses EPA to help shift the eicosanoid balance in the favorable direction. EPA helps dampen inflammation and improves circulation by preventing platelets from sticking together. EPA also lowers cholesterol and especially triglyceride levels and smoothes the heart rhythm. If fish isn't your favorite dish, taking a fish oil supplement is another convenient way to help maintain the proper balance of fats in your body.

Trans Fatty Acids: Unnatural and Unhealthy

The one form of unsaturated fat that you should definitely steer clear of is trans fat. Trans fatty acids are formed whenever vegetable oils are heated to high temperatures. These chemically altered fats are found in foods fried in vegetable oils as well as in packaged foods containing hydrogenated or partially hydrogenated vegetable oils, such as cookies, crackers, bakery products, and some margarines. Though they are unsaturated, trans fatty acids have the same straight configuration as saturated fatty acids—and the same negative effects on health. Trans fatty acids are linked to increased levels of LDL cholesterol, decreased levels of beneficial HDL cholesterol, and an increased risk of cancer, diabetes, and obesity.

Figure 22. A trans fatty acid.

Elaidic acid, found in foods containing partially hydrogenated oils, has the identical chemical formula as the monounsaturated fatty acid oleic acid, but it lacks oleic acid's U-shaped structure. Its straight configuration resembles that of a saturated fatty acid, and it acts much like a saturated fatty acid in your body.

Trans fatty acids are such a significant health risk that, beginning in 2006, the Food and Drug Administration will require that food labels list trans fatty acid content. Until then, the easiest way to avoid these fats is to stay away from fried foods, as well as all packaged foods that contain hydrogenated or partially hydrogenated vegetable oils.

Protein Power

Protein is the substance of which we are made. With the exception of water, protein is the most abundant substance in the body and accounts for up to half of your dry body weight. Proteins are essential components of muscle, skin, hair, and nails, as well as structural ingredients of enzymes, hemoglobin, and immune cells. Amino acids, the building blocks of proteins, are used to make neurotransmitters, the brain's chemical messengers, and some actually serve as neurotransmitters in their own right.

The crucial role that proteins play in the structures of the body is one reason why my version of the Food Pyramid (see page 153) contains protein as the second tier, just above vegetables and fruits. Another reason is that eating protein along with carbohydrates is crucial to keeping insulin levels in the low normal range and preventing you from experiencing the "blood sugar blues" a few hours after eating.

Every meal you eat should contain a serving of protein. Keep in mind that a serving of protein is *not* a quarter-pounder with cheese. For animal protein, a serving is about the size of a deck of cards; for plant protein, roughly the size of a tennis ball. Choose lean meat and poultry like skinless chicken, turkey, or veal; cold-water fish such as salmon, mackerel, or trout; or plant sources such as soy foods or legumes. Egg whites and nonfat or low-fat dairy products are other good choices.

Minimize your intake of egg yolks, organ meats, and high-fat red meat, all of which are concentrated sources of a fatty acid called arachidonic acid (AA). AA is like EPA's evil twin: it essentially reverses the benefits of EPA by fueling inflammation, suppressing immune function, promoting the formation of blood clots, and triggering allergies and skin disorders.

A WARNING ABOUT SUGAR SUBSTITUTES

Most individuals with a weight problem have resorted to consuming sugar substitutes and diet drinks. The most commonly used sugar substitute is aspartame, which can be found in such products as NutraSweet and Equal. Most diet drinks and packaged diet foods also contain aspartame. This represents a dangerous, though largely unrecognized, health risk.

Aspartame is an unnatural substance produced by a large chemical manufacturer. It is a neurotoxin that destroys brain cells. The body breaks down aspartame into formaldehyde, the chemical used by morticians for embalming. Formaldehyde is a known cancer-causing agent. The use of aspartame has been associated with more than 150 symptoms, including increased incidence of brain tumors, mood disorders, declining mental function, and migraine headaches, to name just a few. Over 80 percent of the complaints received by the FDA about food product reactions are related to aspartame. Why hasn't it been taken off the market? Just follow the money trail. The production and sales of aspartame is a multibillion dollar business.

There is a more recent sugar substitute on the market, Splenda (sucralose). Sucralose is also an unnatural substance and is chemically synthesized by adding chlorine molecules to sugar. Chlorinated hydrocarbons found in the petrochemical industry are known carcinogens. Sucralose is a chlorinated hydrocarbon.

An interesting finding in numerous medical studies indicates that unnatural sugar substitutes are associated with weight gain. How many thin people do you know who drink diet sodas and use unnatural sugar substitutes?

My strong recommendation is that you avoid both aspartame and sucralose in all of their forms and use only naturally occurring sugar substitutes.

Two safe sugar substitutes are Xylitol and Stevia, both of which are safe, naturally occurring sweeteners, extracted from certain species of plants.

A FINAL WORD

By implementing the recommendations that I made in chapter 10 and in this appendix, you will have placed yourself on the path leading to optimal health and an ideal body weight.

Appendix C
More About Vitamins and Minerals

In chapter 11, I discussed the importance of a consistent vitamin and mineral supplementation program. Volumes have been written on this subject by such renowned authors such as Adele Davis, Dr. Earl Mindell, Dr. Julian Whitaker, Robert Crayhon, and numerous others.

In this appendix, I will discuss the basic actions of key vitamins and minerals and explain their benefits.

Slow the Aging Process with Antioxidants

The free-radical theory is widely accepted as one explanation of the causes of the degenerative diseases associated with aging. Free radicals are negatively charged molecules that circulate throughout the body, causing damage to the DNA in your cells, leading to cancer and degenerative disease, such as hardening of the arteries, heart disease, Alzheimer's, arthritis, and inflammatory diseases. These free radicals are unstable, highly reactive molecules and are a byproduct of normal cellular activity. Free radicals cause oxidation in our tissues. Oxidation is the same process that causes iron to rust and oil to become rancid in the presence of oxygen. In the same way, our bodies' tissues and organs corrode over time due to the oxidizing effects of free radicals.

Exposure to cigarette smoke, chemicals, radiation, pesticides, and other toxic substances such as drugs are major sources of free radicals that accelerate the aging process. It's important to do all you can to minimize your exposure to them. However, even elements that we think of as benign or beneficial, such as the air we breathe and the food that nourishes us, subject our cells to free radicals. In fact, the majority of free radicals in the body are actually produced within the body during respiration and the breakdown of food into energy.

Fortunately, nature has provided a way to slow the free radical, or oxidative process: antioxidants. Antioxidants are substances such as certain vitamins, minerals, herbs, amino acids, and enzymes that neutralize free radicals in our bodies. Your body produces numerous antioxidants, including the enzymes superoxide dismutase and glutathione peroxidase. However, as we get older, production of these enzymes slows down and our bodies become less effective at neutralizing free radicals. In order to protect yourself from the adverse effect of free radicals and tip the scales in favor of the antioxidants, it is important for you to eat foods rich in antioxidants, such as carrots, broccoli, tomatoes, and green vegetables. It is equally important to bolster your diet with copious amounts of antioxidant supplements, especially vitamin C, vitamin E, Coenzyme Q10, selenium, and zinc.

VITAMIN C BOOSTS IMMUNE FUNCTION

Vitamin C is the premier antioxidant in the water portion of your body. Because your body is 60 percent water, that covers a lot of territory.

Vitamin C's antioxidant powers are important to building a strong immune system. Vitamin C shields DNA from damage that can lead to cancer, increases levels of the anticancer and antiviral chemical interferon, and raises tissue levels of glutathione, one of your body's most important naturally occurring antioxidants. Vitamin C is abundant in the white blood cells that engulf and destroy bacteria and protects these cells from being damaged during this process.

Vitamin C is also the predominant antioxidant in the airways, which is why I insist that my patients with allergies and asthma take high-dose vitamin C. Not only does this vitamin help protect the lungs from the massive onslaught of free radicals that occurs during the allergic response but it also acts as a natural antihistamine.

The only mammals that do not make their own vitamin C are humans, monkeys, and guinea pigs. All other mammals make 6,000 mg of vitamin C per 150 pounds of body weight. Humans must obtain vitamin C from food or supplements. Because the therapeutic benefits of vitamin C are so well documented, I recommend that my adult patients supplement with 6,000 mg of vitamin C per day and that they double this amount if they are sick. Large amounts of vitamin C may lead to loose stools which can be easily corrected by reducing daily intake by one fourth.

VITAMIN E PROTECTS YOUR HEART

The star antioxidant in the lipid, or fat, portion of your tissues, is vitamin E. Did you know that cardiologists are five times more likely than their patients to take vitamin E? That's probably because cardiologists are aware that vitamin E works on many fronts to stave off heart disease. For starters, it protects LDL cholesterol from oxidation. This is crucial, since only oxidized LDL cholesterol, which has taken a "hit" from a free radical, poses a threat to the health of arteries. In its oxidized form, LDL cholesterol readily adheres to artery walls, contributing to the formation of plaques that eventually stiffen and narrow the arteries and increase the risk of heart attack and stroke.

Vitamin E also enhances blood flow, helps prevent blood clots, counters inflammation, and protects the endothelium, the inner lining of the artery, which is especially vulnerable to free-radical damage. All of these benefits add up to a significant reduction in heart disease risk with supplemental vitamin E. In the Cambridge Heart Antioxidant Study (CHAOS), a double-blind, placebo-controlled study of over two thousand adults, those who took 400–800 IU of vitamin E per day had 77-percent fewer heart attacks than the placebo group over a sixteen-month period.

But vitamin E has more wide-ranging benefits. It is the most prevalent antioxidant in the fatty tissues of your body, including the membranes that surround each and every one of your cells. Just as the walls of a fortress are the first-line defense against invasion by the enemy, cell membranes are the primary barrier keeping toxins and other harmful chemicals from entering the cell and damaging DNA. Vitamin E is actually incorporated into cell membranes, where it protects against damage from lead and other heavy metals, pesticides and other poisons, and free radicals generated within your own body.

The RDA for vitamin E is a mere 15 mg, approximately 22 IU per day. But because the research on high-dose vitamin E is so compelling, I recommend taking 800 IU per day. You simply cannot get this amount of vitamin E from food, unless you want to eat over a thousand almonds at one sitting. The simplest, healthiest way to get a therapeutic dose of vitamin E is to take a high-potency nutritional supplement.

Support Your Heart With Coenzyme Q10

Coenzyme Q10 (CoQ10) is an integral part of the mitochondria, the engine of your cells where the energy is generated to run your body. Organs such as the heart, liver, kidneys, spleen, and pancreas, which require large amounts of energy, need high levels of CoQ10. As you age, your CoQ10 levels fall. Studies indicate that when levels of CoQ10 decline by 25 percent, your organs cannot meet their energy requirements and major health problems can result. The statin cholesterol lowering drugs such as Zocor, Lipitor, Pravachol, and Crestor, deplete CoQ10 levels and are associated with numerous side effects. I recommend that my patients take 120 mg of CoQ10 per day. Anyone taking statin drugs should take twice this amount.

Cut Cancer Risk With Selenium

Selenium is considered a trace mineral because it is present in the body in a nearly infinitesimal amount—a mere two-hundredths of a gram, compared to the 1,150 grams of calcium that are found in the body. But don't be fooled by this statistic into thinking that selenium isn't important. This mighty mineral is a powerful antioxidant and a valuable weapon in the fight against cancer. Selenium enables your cells to convert the inactive thyroid hormone T4 to the active thyroid hormone T3.

Selenium protects against cancer in four ways. First, it directly repairs the free-radical damage to DNA that initiates and promotes cancer. Second, when cells do mutate, selenium triggers apoptosis, or programmed cell death, preventing out-of-control growth of malignant cells. Third, selenium functions as part of the antioxidant and detoxifying agent glutathione. Fourth, selenium enhances your cells' ability to utilize thyroid hormone.

A number of studies show that low selenium levels carry with them an increased risk of cancer. The reverse is also true: taking a selenium supplement can be highly protective against cancer. In a study of patients with a history of skin cancer, those who were given 200 mcg of selenium per day—almost four times the RDA—had a 37-percent reduced risk of cancer compared to those who received a placebo. Their risk of lung cancer was reduced by 45 percent, colorectal cancer risk was cut by 58 percent, and prostate cancer risk was reduced by 63 percent. In fact, the supplement takers showed such a dramatic decrease in cancer incidence that the researchers halted the study two years early because they felt it was unethical to deprive the placebo group of the benefits of this mineral.

To get the maximum protection from this cancer-fighting antioxidant, I recommend taking 400 mcg of selenium per day.

ZINC ADDS ZIP TO IMMUNE FUNCTION

Zinc participates in more enzymatic reactions than any other mineral, including chemical reactions needed to make DNA and RNA and to synthesize proteins. Zinc is necessary for the proper action of the sex hormones, thyroid hormones, and growth hormone and for the conversion of vitamin A to its active form.

Optimal immune function requires zinc, which has direct antiviral effects and supports the activity of white blood cells. Zinc deficiency makes infections more likely, including infections of the digestive tract that can cause further nutritional deficiencies. Because zinc is essential to the formation of proteins, low zinc levels can impair wound healing.

Zinc deficiency is quite common, since average intakes of zinc are half to two-thirds of the recommended amount. I recommend supplementing with 10 to 20 mg per day of zinc.

Besides the key antioxidants that I have just described, allow me to recommend some additional vitamins and minerals which can be beneficial to your health.

"B" SMART: TAKE B COMPLEX

Not too long ago, the cholesterol theory of heart disease ruled. High cholesterol was considered the major culprit in heart disease, despite the fact that 50 percent of those who suffer heart attacks have total cholesterol levels in the "normal" range, below 200 mg/dL. But in recent years, the so-called cholesterol theory has grown considerably more complicated as new risk factors for heart disease have been identified. One of the most important may be elevated levels of homocysteine. In the Physicians' Health Study, a long-term study involving almost fifteen thousand male physicians, men with the highest homocysteine levels had a threefold higher risk of heart disease compared to those with lower levels.

Homocysteine is a toxic byproduct of the breakdown of methionine, an essential amino acid found in meat and other protein-rich foods. When homocysteine accumulates in your tissues, it wreaks havoc with the functioning of cells. In addition to dramatically increasing the risk of heart attack, high levels of homocysteine are linked to an increased risk of stroke, Alzheimer's disease, depression, osteoporosis, and certain types of cancer.

Fortunately, your body has an efficient system for detoxifying homocysteine called methylation. Methylation essentially reverses the process of homocysteine production by transforming this toxin back into methionine. Methylation is such a crucial "housekeeping" procedure that defects in this process are considered to be a key factor in aging.

At least two B vitamins are essential participants in the methylation process—vitamin B_{12} and folic acid—and blood levels of these nutrients show an inverse relationship with homocysteine levels. In other words, the lower your B_{12} and folic acid levels, the higher your homocysteine is likely to be—and the greater your risk of heart disease. Heart disease is the number one cause of death in America. The good news is that by boosting your levels of B_{12} and folic acid you can reduce your risk of heart disease. In the Nurses' Health Study, the female counterpart of the Physicians' Health Study, women with the highest intake of folic acid had a 31-percent lower risk of heart attack compared to those with the lowest intake. Analysts have calculated that if every man and woman of middle age or older received folic acid and vitamin B_{12} supplements, health care costs would be reduced by more than \$2 billion over a ten-year period. And think of all the lives that would be saved!

Vitamin B_{12} and folic acid should always be supplemented together, because each depends on the other for activation. Actually, all of the B vitamins interact in complex ways, both among themselves and with other nutrients. Without vitamin B_2 (riboflavin), the activity of vitamin B_6 (pyridoxine) is impaired. And without vitamin B_6, calcium absorption is impaired. Furthermore, virtually all of the B vitamins are essential to the enzymatic reactions that release energy from carbohydrates, fats, and proteins, and a deficiency of any one of them can bring the entire metabolic process to a halt.

This is the bottom line. Look for a supplement that contains all of the B complex vitamins, and make sure it contains at least 60 mcg of vitamin B_{12} and 400 mcg of folic acid.

Vitamin D: Are You Deficient?

Even in Texas, where I live, there is significantly less sunlight in the winter months. For some, the decline in sunlight brings on seasonal affective disorder, or "the winter blues." But for all of us, it brings the risk of low vitamin D levels because our primary source of vitamin D is exposure to sunlight.

Vitamin D's most important role is to facilitate calcium absorption from the intestines into the bones. Not surprisingly, the classic vitamin D deficiency disease is a bone-softening disease of childhood called rickets. Before the fortification of milk and other dairy products with vitamin D, rickets was quite prevalent, especially in the northern latitudes. Today, it is a relatively rare disease in this country.

However, at the other end of the age spectrum, vitamin D deficiency remains a serious problem, especially among nursing home residents and the housebound elderly. Adults who avoid dairy products due to lactose intolerance and those with kidney disease or intestinal problems that impair absorption are also at greater risk. But even those without obvious risk factors who consume the RDA for vitamin D may be deficient. In a study of adults admitted to a medical ward at Massachusetts General Hospital, 57 percent were deficient in vitamin D—including 43 percent of those whose intake of vitamin D was above the RDA. These were not elderly individuals, but adults of all ages.

The most dramatic effect of vitamin D deficiency in adults is osteomalacia, the adult version of rickets. But vitamin D deficiency is also linked to impaired immunity, mood disorders, hypertension, and an increased risk of cancer of the breast, ovary, prostate, and colon. It can hasten the progression of arthritis, reduce resistance to infection, and worsen insulin resistance.

I recommend getting a minimum of fifteen minutes of sunscreen-free exposure to the sun at least three times a week. Darker-skinned individuals will need at least twice this amount. In addition, I recommend supplementing with 300–400 IU of vitamin D daily.

Bone Up on Calcium

Everyone knows that calcium helps build strong bones. But did you know that calcium helps regulate your heartbeat? Calcium is also required for normal blood clotting, contraction of your muscles, transmission of nerve impulses, and secretion of some hormones.

Many Americans fail to get enough calcium from their diet. In a recent national survey, researchers found that men over age sixty who did not take calcium supplements consumed only 61 percent of the recommended amount of calcium per day. Women over age sixty—the population at greatest risk of osteoporosis— fared even worse, consuming just 48 percent of the recommended amount from food and dairy products.

But inadequate consumption of calcium is only half of the problem. The other half is excessive consumption of foods and beverages that actually promote calcium loss. A high-protein diet is one factor that contributes to calcium excretion, as is excessive sodium intake. However, the greatest contributor to calcium loss in this country is likely to be our addiction to coffee and other caffeinated beverages. Colas are especially harmful because they contain not just one but two calcium-depleting chemicals: caffeine and phosphoric acid.

Taking supplemental calcium is a simple way to ensure you're getting enough of this important mineral. Research shows that supplemental calcium not only reduces the risk of bone fracture, but also protects against some types of cancer. In a five-year study of over 125,000 men and women, those who took at least 500 mg of supplemental calcium had a 31-percent lower risk of colorectal cancer than those who took no calcium supplements.

I recommend supplementing with a minimum of 1,000 mg per day of calcium. For maximum absorption, choose calcium citrate or calcium chelate rather than calcium carbonate. Calcium and magnesium should always be taken together in a two-to-one ratio of calcium to magnesium. In other words, for every 1,000 mg of calcium you take, you should take 500 mg of magnesium. Women with osteopenia or osteoporosis should take upwards of 2,000 mg of calcium per day, again balanced with magnesium in a two-to-one ratio.

MAGNESIUM IS A MUST

Though magnesium is not as popular a supplement as calcium, it deserves to be. A full 40 percent of your bone mass is accounted for by magnesium, and it is as important as calcium for preventing osteoporosis.

But magnesium's benefits extend beyond your bones. This mineral supports healthy respiratory function by helping to relax the bronchial smooth muscles. Asthma sufferers are commonly deficient in magnesium, and this alone can trigger an asthma attack. The reverse is also true. Studies have shown that intravenous magnesium can halt an acute asthma attack, while smaller doses taken orally can lessen the likelihood of future attacks.

Magnesium is also good preventive medicine for any type of heart condition. It helps correct irregular heart rhythms, lowers blood pressure, reduces the frequency of angina, and even protects the heart from damage following a heart attack. I wish I had known about the incredible therapeutic benefits of magnesium when my father's heart was damaged on the operating table in 1988. I would have insisted he receive intravenous magnesium to help his heart recover from the devastating effects of that surgical catastrophe.

Deficiencies of magnesium are quite common, especially among the elderly and in women during the premenstrual period. Many drugs reduce magnesium levels, including diuretics and oral contraceptives. I recommend that everyone supplement with 500 mg of magnesium per day.

Potassium and Sodium: Dynamic Duo

Potassium and sodium are the Fred Astaire and Ginger Rogers of minerals. These two minerals perform an intricate dance across cell membranes, creating an electrical potential that fires nerve impulses and muscular contractions. The proper balance of these minerals is crucial to maintaining the right fluid volume inside cells as well as for regulating blood pressure and heartbeat.

An excess of sodium can contribute to high blood pressure, heart disease, and stroke. If you have asthma, too much sodium can increase your sensitivity to allergens. A high-sodium diet has even been linked to a greater risk of osteoporosis. On the other hand, an increased intake of potassium can help lower blood pressure, reduce the risk of heart attack and stroke, and even improve insulin sensitivity.

Unfortunately, most of us get too much sodium and too little potassium in our diet. While the optimal balance of potassium to sodium is at least 5:1 (5 mg of potassium for every 1 mg of sodium), most of us have a potassium-to-sodium ratio of 1:2 or even worse. There are two reasons for this huge imbalance: we eat too many high-sodium processed foods and too few potassium-rich fresh fruits and vegetables.

Fruits and vegetables in their natural state have a potassium-to-sodium ratio of at least 50:1—and for some, it's as high as 500:1. As foods are processed, sodium is added and potassium is lost, shifting the ratio in the other direction. At least 75 percent of the sodium we consume comes not from the saltshaker but from sodium added to foods by manufacturers during processing. Unless you check the label, it's sometimes hard to detect high levels of sodium because many foods with a high sodium content don't taste salty at all. For example, you may be surprised to learn that cornflakes and instant pudding contain more sodium per serving than salted peanuts.

The bottom line: do everything you can to reduce your intake of high-sodium processed foods while stepping up your consumption of potassium-rich fresh vegetables and fruits. To help shift your potassium-to-sodium ratio back in the positive direction, I also recommend supplementing with 200 mg of potassium per day.

As a medical doctor, I am convinced about the absolute need for and benefits of vitamin and mineral supplementation. The vitamins and minerals that I have discussed above are the basics and should be included in your daily health regimen. They have been in mine since 1989. There are many other supplements that I personally use and recommend to my patients. For additional information about vitamins and minerals, I recommend that you peruse the titles of the books in appendix G and obtain one for your study.

Appendix D
Yeast-Free Eating and Beyond

If your score on the Yeast Overgrowth Questionnaire indicates a candida problem, then I recommend that you follow the three-step program I outlined in chapter 5 to eradicate yeast, eliminate foods that contain or nourish yeast, and repopulate your gastrointestinal tract with friendly bacteria.

Eradication of yeast (step one) is best done using the antifungal preparations nystatin and Diflucan (fluconazole). However, these drugs are available by prescription only. If your doctor is not willing to prescribe these drugs, another option is to add garlic to your diet or take garlic capsules. Garlic is a natural antifungal that can help prevent and treat yeast overgrowth.

The most challenging part of this program is eliminating dietary sources of yeast and foods that allow yeast to thrive (step two). Though the yeast-free, grain-free eating program may seem like a difficult regimen to follow, keep in mind that you only have to adhere to it for thirty days. It will help if you focus on all the foods that are permitted rather than on the foods that must be avoided for this time period.

Repopulation of beneficial bacteria (step three) can be accomplished easily by taking a probiotic supplement. Probiotics are "friendly" bacteria such as *Lactobacillus acidophilus* and *Bifidobacterium bifidum* that normally inhabit the colon, helping to keep candida in check.

Here is everything you need to know in order to follow the thirty-day yeast-free, grain-free eating program.

The following foods are permitted during the thirty-day yeast-free, grain-free period:

- Meats (chicken, beef, turkey, pork, lamb, venison, and seafood)
- Vegetables (limit starchy vegetables such as squash, corn, carrots)
- Salads
- Dried beans (black, red, and kidney beans)
- Eggs (boiled, poached, scrambled, or fried with olive oil)
- Oatmeal (slow-cooking; in recipes only)
- Lemons and limes
- Avocados
- Black olives
- Cold-pressed olive oil
- Nuts and nut butters (without added sugar)
- Herbal teas
- Coffee and tea (not decaffeinated)
- Xylitol (a natural caloric sweetener; can be used in beverages and recipes that call for sugar)

After two weeks, you may add the following foods:
- Fruits (with the exception of fruit juice, grapes, and bananas)
- Butter

During the thirty-day yeast-free, grain-free period, avoid the following:

- Sugar (check labels for dextrose, sucrose, fructose, lactose, maltose, maltodextrin, cane sugar, beet sugar, honey, corn syrup, high-fructose corn syrup, fruit juice concentrate, maple syrup or solids, and molasses)
- Artificial sweeteners such as aspartame, saccharin, and sucralose are never recommended.
- Fruit juices, grapes, and bananas
- Milk and milk products (cheese, yogurt, sour cream, ice cream, and milk-based dressings)
- Breads and baked goods (cereals, crackers, biscuits, rolls, and flour tortillas)
- Grains (corn, wheat, rye, millet, rice, and barley)
- Pasta
- Potatoes
- Mushrooms
- Soft drinks (including sugar-free soft drinks) and decaffeinated beverages
- Alcohol
- Vinegar and products containing vinegar (pickles, green olives, salad dressings, soy sauce, mustard, mayonnaise, ketchup, salsa, etc.)
- Vegetable shortening, margarine, and partially hydrogenated oils are never recommended.

ON YOUR MARK

1. Take inventory of foods at home. To avoid temptation, throw out or give away any "forbidden" foods.

2. Prepare a shopping list and menu plans for the week.

3. Buy your groceries for the week.
    a. Purchase fresh deli meat from the deli counter (no prepackaged deli meats). Purchase a pound of each type of meat (roast beef, ham, chicken, and turkey) to enable you to rotate your foods. This is an easy way to get protein with your snacks and meals, especially if you are on the go.
    b. Fresh vegetables are healthiest. Frozen are second best, and canned are a distant third. If you do buy frozen or canned vegetables, read the labels carefully. Avoid any products with added sugar.
    c. Avoid packaged foods as much as possible, as they tend to contain a multitude of hidden additives and ingredients. If you do purchase packaged foods, read labels carefully before buying. Search the ingredient list for yeast, sugar in all its disguises (see list on previous page), vinegar, dairy products, vegetable shortening, margarine, and partially hydrogenated oils.
    d. Purchase xylitol to be used as your sweetener.

4. If your doctor has prescribed nystatin and Diflucan (fluconazole) to eradicate yeast, fill your prescriptions in advance. Otherwise, purchase fresh garlic to be used liberally throughout

the month, or purchase a garlic supplement to be taken daily. Also, purchase a high-quality probiotic supplement. To help with yeast "die-off," purchase baking soda (sodium bicarbonate) or Alka-Seltzer Gold.

5. Pick a "start day," write it on your calendar, and stick to it.

6. Find a friend or family member to join you or hold you accountable during your new eating program. This will help you be more successful. Also, inform your coworkers, family members and friends about the eating program and what is involved. They can be your supporters.

Get Set

1. Cut up fresh vegetables for snacks or steaming with meals. (Keep in sealed plastic bags or containers.) Do this after each shopping trip.

2. Boil a dozen eggs for a quick and easy snack or breakfast protein. Refrigerate.

3. Prepare recipes for condiments, salad dressings, and sauces. (See recipes in appendix E.)

4. Each evening, remove frozen meats and place in refrigerator for thawing.

5. You may want to sort your medications and supplements in a daily pill organizer so that you don't forget to take them each day.

Go!

1. Rotate all foods. Don't get into the habit of eating the same foods day after day, as this is one way that food allergies develop. Use a menu planner to ensure that you rotate your foods. (See "Food Rotation" on page 247 for guidelines.)

2. When cooking your meals, plan to make enough for leftovers. Use leftovers in your meals the next day.

3. Steam vegetables or eat them raw. This is much more nutritious than boiling the vitamins out of the vegetables.

4. Meats should be broiled, baked, or grilled. Microwaving is acceptable but do not fry meats.

5. Be creative by adding new spices to enhance the flavor of both vegetables and meats. Most seasonings are acceptable, but make sure that the seasoning contains no added sugar or dairy products such as dried milk or Parmesan, and try to avoid MSG.

6. Do not hesitate to alter the ingredients of your favorite recipes; remove all the "restricted" ingredients and substitute with other "safe" ingredients.

    a. For any recipe that requires vinegar, substitute with

an equal amount of lemon juice (fresh or concentrated).

b. Instead of using butter as a sauce for vegetables or meat marinades, use cold-pressed olive oil and your favorite spice. Chicken broth can also be used in place of butter when making sauces.

c. Use xylitol instead of sugar in beverages and recipes that call for sugar.

d. Substitute soy or oat milk in any recipe calling for cream or milk.

e. Substitute soy or oat flour in the place of any other flours.

f. Do not use store-bought sauces (barbecue sauce, salad dressings, Worcestershire sauce, soy sauce, etc.). Instead, make your own sauces. (See appendix E.)

g. Egg substitute can be used in place of whole eggs, if desired.

7. Never skip breakfast. All meals are important, but breakfast is critical because it determines your metabolism for the rest of the day. Any time you skip a meal, you will be setting yourself up to cheat. Throw out the idea of a conventional breakfast. Try broiled meats and vegetables in the morning.

8. Drink at least eight 8-ounce glasses of water daily. This detoxifies the body of yeast and lessens food allergy reactions.

9. Review your social/personal calendar for upcoming events (weddings, showers, dinner parties, etc.) and preplan your meals. Inquire about what is being served, and if no "safe" foods are available, bring your own foods if possible or eat beforehand. Choose restaurants that can accommodate your needs.

10. Remember that the closer you follow the eating program, the better you will feel.

Hints for Yeast-Free Dining

It is possible to enjoy some of your favorite restaurants while on the yeast-free eating program. It will require discipline, planning, and a willingness to ask questions. As long as you remember to adhere to all the rules of the yeast-free eating program, you will be surprised to discover the wonderful meals you can still enjoy. Here are some helpful hints:

1. Preplan! Make a list of the restaurants you enjoy, then determine if they serve foods within the program, such as grilled chicken (without a sauce), fajita meat (minus the tortilla), and steamed vegetables. Remember, stay away from pastas, breads, and processed salad dressings.

2. Be disciplined! If possible, decide what you will order before arriving at the restaurant. If you try to decide once you get there, you may be tempted to order dishes that are counterproductive to the program.

3. Ask questions! Do not be afraid to ask questions of your waiter or other restaurant staff. They should be able to answer questions pertaining to the menu.

4. Request substitutions! Most fine restaurants accept special requests. Politely ask if substitutions can be made to a menu item if there are no appropriate entrees. For salads, make your own dressing at the table using fresh lemons, cold-pressed olive oil, salt, and pepper.

5. Be creative! Try foods you have never tried before. You may discover some new, healthy favorites.

6. Be in control! Ask your waiter NOT to bring the bread, chips, wine list, or dessert tray to your table. Having these items on your table will only be a temptation.

7. Keep it simple! Stick to the basics, such as grilled or baked chicken, steak, lobster, shrimp, turkey, steamed vegetables, and dinner salads with your own dressing. Avoid casseroles, sauces, and breaded or fried foods. These foods tend to have hidden ingredients.

AT THE FINISH LINE

After completing one month on the yeast-free eating program you should conduct an oral challenge to yeast. Here's how to do it:

Eat two pieces of whole wheat bread with a glass of water. Monitor your symptoms for one hour. If no symptoms develop, then perform a second challenge by eating two additonal pieces of whole wheat bread with a glass of water. DO NOT have any more yeast products for two days and watch for delayed symptoms. If no symptoms occur, then you may add yeast products back into your diet in moderation. If symptoms do occur, then eliminate yeast products for another month. (For a list of symptoms, see the "Test Yourself for Yeast Overgrowth" questionnaire, appendix A.)

HAPPY TRAILS

If you want to continue on the yeast-free, grain-free eating program, rest assured that it is a healthy diet that can safely be followed for as long as you choose to do so. It is an ideal eating program for anyone with diabetes, hypoglycemia, elevated cholesterol and/or triglycerides, or heart disease, as well as for anyone who wants to experience better health and a strong immune system.

If you do want to reintroduce some of the foods that were excluded from the yeast-free, grain-free eating program, go slowly! Add one food group at a time. For example, add products containing vinegar for three days and note any symptoms that arise. (See "The Oral Food Challenge" below for guidelines on managing symptoms.) If you tolerate these foods, add dairy products for three days and note any symptoms that arise.

Whatever you do, continue to avoid sugar and yeast as much as possible. This will help keep candida at bay and prevent you from experiencing sugar highs and lows.

The Oral Food Challenge

The oral food challenge is a simple way to confirm or disprove a food allergy. Though skin testing is helpful to identify food allergies, some foods that provoke a skin response do not always cause an internal response. It is the internal response that is of concern, and the simplest way to identify internal symptoms is by undergoing an oral food challenge.

The oral food challenge is also helpful to identify masked food allergies. A masked food allergy is one in which the symptoms are not immediate or obvious. Ingesting the problem food may provide temporary relief of symptoms, so when the symptoms recur, you may find yourself being drawn again to that food. Over time, you may need to eat more of the food to keep the symptoms at bay. For this reason, masked food allergies are sometimes called food addictions.

HOW TO PERFORM THE ORAL FOOD CHALLENGE:

1. Choose which ONE food you will challenge.

2. Eat this food every day for four consecutive days (at least one serving per day). If severe symptoms occur, then the food may be discontinued.

3. Avoid this food for the next four consecutive days. Be sure to omit both the food and any products containing the food as an ingredient for this four-day period.

4. On the morning of the ninth day, eat a portion of the food with nothing but a glass of water. Watch for symptoms over the next hour. If no symptoms occur, eat a second portion of the food with nothing but a glass of water. Continue to monitor for symptoms for the next three days, but do not eat any more of this food.

5. A food (in antigen form) stays in the body for approximately seventy-two hours, so you may experience a reaction up to three days after eating a particular food. A food reaction can affect virtually any part of the body. You may notice aching joints, diarrhea, constipation, headaches, irritability, depressed moods, marked fatigue, nervousness, anxiety, difficulty concentrating, allergy symptoms (sneezing, postnasal drainage, cough, ringing ears, watery eyes, etc.), hives/itching/rash, cramps/bloating/gas, asthma or breathing difficulty, canker sores, or an exacerbation of current symptoms.

6. If you do react to a food, baking soda or Alka-Seltzer Gold may help neutralize your reaction.

7. If you experience a mild reaction to the food, you may choose to keep the food in your diet on a five-day rotation plan. However, a better tactic is avoidance. If you faithfully avoid the problem food for six months to two years, you can generally eliminate the food allergy, which will allow you to bring the food back into the diet on a rotated basis.

8. For moderate to severe reactions, the best tactic is avoidance. Strict avoidance may eventually enable you to reintroduce the food on a rotated basis, unless it is a fixed food allergy. The most common foods causing fixed allergies are peanuts, strawberries, and shellfish. Food allergy drops may be of benefit for foods that are difficult to avoid such as wheat, corn, eggs, milk, and soy. However, food drops will neutralize your reaction to the food only for a twenty-four-hour time period. They will not eliminate the allergy.

FOOD ROTATION

Repetitious eating is the number one cause of food allergies. The body becomes overloaded with a particular food and begins to make antibodies against that food. This results in adverse symptoms and presents the body with one more allergen to combat. Repeatedly putting the offending food into the body further taxes the immune system.

Following a rotation diet is the best way to avoid overloading your body with a particular food and developing a food allergy. Remember, a food stays in the body in antigen form for three days. To avoid repeating a food in close succession, a five-day rotation diet is best. This requires a bit of preplanning to rotate each food category through a five-day cycle. For example, for meats, you might have beef on Monday, chicken on Tuesday, seafood on Wednesday, pork on Thursday, and turkey on Friday, beginning a new five-day cycle on Saturday. You would do the same for vegetables, fruits, and other food items.

Eating for Energy

Whether you're adhering to the yeast-free, grain-free diet or not, it's important to follow the principles of healthy eating outlined in chapter 10. To maximize energy throughout the day and minimize the "blood sugar blues," be sure to eat three meals a day and balance your protein and carbohydrate intake at every meal. To review, divide your plate into three sections. The first section will contain a serving of protein (for animal sources, about the size of a deck of cards; for plant sources, roughly the size of a tennis ball), the second will contain a serving of vegetables (about the size of your fist), and the third will contain a serving of fruit (again, about the size of your fist). Include some healthy monounsaturated fats from olives, nuts, or avocados, and be sure to drink a full glass of water before every meal.

To select the healthiest sources of protein, carbohydrates, and fats, refer to the charts that follow. Proteins and fats are categorized as favorable (appropriate for frequent consumption), fair (enjoy in moderation), or poor (eat only occasionally). For vegetables and fruits, there are only two categories: favorable (appropriate for frequent consumption) and poor (eat only occasionally).

Favorable Proteins
- Chicken breast, no skin
- Eggs
- Seafood
- Turkey breast
- Veal
- Venison

Fair Proteins
- Beef, lean cuts
- Canadian bacon, lean
- Chicken, dark, no skin
- Corned beef, lean
- Duck
- Ham, deli style
- Ham, lean
- Lamb, lean
- Pork, lean
- Pork chop
- Soy products
- Turkey, dark, no skin
- Turkey bacon
- Tofu

Poor Proteins
- Bacon
- Beef, fatty cuts
- Beef, ground
- Bologna
- Hot dogs (any meat)
- Kielbasa
- Liver
- Pepperoni
- Pork sausage
- Salami

Favorable Vegetables and Legumes
- Artichoke
- Asparagus
- Bean sprouts
- Black beans
- Bok choy
- Broccoli
- Brussels sprouts
- Cabbage
- Cauliflower
- Celery
- Collard greens
- Cucumber
- Eggplant
- Garbanzo beans
- Green pepper
- Green/wax beans
- Kale
- Kidney beans
- Leeks

- Lentils
- Lettuce
- Okra
- Onions
- Radishes
- Spaghetti squash
- Spinach
- Swiss chard
- Tomato
- Turnip greens
- Turnips
- Yellow squash
- Zucchini

Poor Vegetables and Legumes

- Acorn squash
- Baked beans
- Beets
- Butternut squash
- Carrots
- Corn
- Lima beans
- Parsnips
- Peas
- Pinto beans, canned
- Potatoes
- Refried beans
- Sweet potatoes

Favorable Fruits
- Apple
- Apricots
- Blackberries
- Blueberries
- Cantaloupe
- Grapefruit
- Honeydew
- Kiwi
- Lemon
- Lime
- Nectarine
- Orange
- Peach
- Pear
- Pineapple
- Plum
- Raspberries
- Strawberries
- Tangerine
- Watermelon

Poor Fruits
- Banana
- Cranberries
- Dates
- Figs
- Fruit juices
- Guava
- Kumquat
- Mango

- Papaya
- Prunes
- Raisins

Favorable Fats
- Almonds
- Avocados
- Canola oil
- Cashews
- Cold-pressed olive oil
- Macadamia nuts
- Olives
- Pecans
- Sunflower seeds

Fair Fats
- Butter
- Sesame oil
- Soybean oil
- Walnuts

Poor Fats
- Cream
- Cream cheese
- Hard cheeses
- Lard
- Margarines containing hydrogenated or partially hydrogenated oil
- Vegetable shortening

APPENDIX E
Recipes

DRESSINGS, SAUCES, AND CONDIMENTS

Avocado & Lemon-Herb Dressing

1 med. avocado, peeled, pitted & quartered
2 cups cold-pressed olive oil
$^1/_2$ cup water
$^1/_4$ cup fresh lemon juice
2 Tbsp. each fresh basil & parsley, chopped
1 Tbsp. each fresh oregano & thyme, chopped
1 Tbsp. tarragon & savory, chopped
1 tsp. each fresh sage & rosemary, chopped
1 tsp. salt

Directions:
Place avocado in a blender or food processor; blend until creamy. Add rest of ingredients; blend until liquid consistency. Pour dressing into a quart jar with a tight-fitting lid; refrigerate until ready to serve.

Basil & Garlic Salad Dressing

1 cup cold-pressed olive oil
$^1/_4$ cup fresh lemon juice
6 stems fresh basil, with leaves
4 large cloves garlic, coarsely chopped
1 tsp. salt

Directions:

Pour olive oil into a 1-cup jar. Scrub basil; pull off leaves from stems and place in oil. Add garlic. Cover with a tight-fitting lid; set on a sunny windowsill for 2–7 days (for more flavor leave longer). Shake container daily; taste for desired flavor. When ready, strain liquid carefully into a measuring cup and discard leaves and garlic. Pour liquid into larger container; add lemon juice and salt, and chill before serving.

Savory Spanish Dressing

1 med. avocado, pitted & peeled
1 large fresh tomato
2 large green onions, peeled
$^1/_2$ tsp. garlic powder
2 Tbsp. fresh lemon juice
$^1/_4$ tsp. cumin
Cayenne pepper to taste

Directions:

Mix all ingredients in a food processor until creamy; pour over salad.

Poppy Seed French Dressing

$^1/_2$ cup cold-pressed olive oil
$^1/_4$ cup fresh lemon juice
1 large clove garlic, minced
$^1/_2$ tsp. salt
$^1/_2$ tsp. fresh basil, chopped
1 tsp. each fresh thyme & tarragon, chopped
$^1/_2$ tsp. ground paprika
$^1/_2$ cup xylitol
$^1/_4$ cup poppy seeds

Directions:
Combine all ingredients in a blender or food processor; mix well. Cover and refrigerate for at least 1 hour before serving.

Creamy Herb Dressing

$^1/_2$ cup cold-pressed olive oil
1 large tomato, quartered
$^1/_4$ cup fresh lemon juice
2 large cloves garlic, crushed
$^1/_2$ tsp. salt
1 Tbsp. each fresh thyme & tarragon, chopped
$^1/_2$ tsp. ground paprika
4 tsp. xylitol
2 Tbsp. sesame seeds

Directions:
Place all ingredients in a blender, food processor, or wide-mouthed jar; mix well. Refrigerate before serving.

Gourmet Sauce

3 Tbsp. cold-pressed olive oil
2 green onions, chopped
1 large clove garlic, minced
$1/2$ tsp. fresh rosemary, chopped
$1/4$ tsp. tarragon

Directions:
Heat oil in a large skillet. Add onions, garlic, rosemary, and tarragon; mix. Simmer 10 minutes or until thoroughly cooked.

Spaghetti Sauce Plus

1 onion, chopped
$1/2$ green bell pepper, chopped
$1/4$ tsp. garlic powder
$1/4$ tsp. pepper
$1/2$–1 tsp. oregano
1 (10 oz.) can tomato paste
1 (10 oz.) can tomato puree
1 large can stewed tomatoes

Directions:
Brown onion, green pepper, garlic powder, pepper, and oregano. Add paste, puree, and tomatoes. Simmer at least $1/2$ hour.

Sauce variations:

With beef: Brown 1 lb. ground meat with onion.

With chicken: Bone chicken breasts. Bread with oat flour. Fry in cold-pressed olive oil on both sides until golden. Pour 1 small can of tomato sauce over top. Bake in shallow pan at 350°F for $1/2$ hour.

Tomato Topping

6 Tbsp. tomato paste
$^1/_4$ cup fresh lemon juice
Chopped fresh oregano & basil to taste
$^1/_4$ tsp. onion powder

Directions:
Mix all ingredients in a small bowl. Serve over meat loaf or choice of dish.

Blender Mayonnaise

6 large egg yolks
2 cups safflower oil or canola oil
$^1/_4$ cup fresh lemon juice
$^1/_4$ cup water
1 tsp. salt
$^1/_4$ tsp. paprika
1 tsp. mustard powder

Directions:
Beat yolks for 2 minutes in a blender. Slowly drizzle 1 cup of oil into the yolks, while beating at a high speed, until all has been used; mixture should become thick. Drizzle in remaining cup, still beating at high speed. Add lemon juice, water, salt, paprika, and mustard powder; mix. Spoon mixture into a widemouthed quart jar with a tight-fitting lid. Refrigerate until ready to use.

Classic Italian Dressing

$^2/_3$ cup cold-pressed olive oil
$^1/_2$ cup fresh lemon juice
$^1/_2$ cup water
2 large cloves garlic, minced
1 Tbsp. each of fresh oregano, basil, & sage
2 Tbsp. xylitol
$^1/_2$ tsp. salt
$^1/_4$ tsp. pepper

Directions:

Combine all ingredients in a small bottle or jar with a tight-fitting lid. Refrigerate for several hours and shake well before serving. Serve over salad or fresh vegetables or use as a marinade.

Mild Mustard

2 tsp. dry mustard powder
1 cup water
3 tsp. arrowroot
$^1/_4$ tsp. turmeric
$^1/_4$ tsp. salt
1 tsp. lemon juice

Directions:

Combine the dry mustard and water in a saucepan and allow them to stand for 10 minutes. Stir in the arrowroot, turmeric, and salt. Heat the mixture over medium heat, stirring often until it thickens and boils. Stir in lemon juice and refrigerate the mustard. Makes about 1 cup.

Homemade Ketchup

4 cups tomato juice
$1/4$ cup lemon juice
2 buds garlic, whole
1 Tbsp. xylitol

Directions:
In a large saucepan, combine tomato juice, lemon juice, and garlic. Bring to a boil, then reduce heat and simmer uncovered for about $2^{1/2}$ hours, until desired thickness. Remove garlic buds and stir in sweetener. Simmer 5 more minutes. Store in refrigerator.

Seafood Cocktail Sauce

1 cup ketchup (see the above recipe)
1 Tbsp. lemon juice

Directions:
Mix ingredients together and chill.

Homemade Guacamole

3 med. ripe avocados, mashed
2 Tbsp. fresh lemon or lime juice
1 large fresh tomato, chopped
3 small green onions, chopped
$^1/_2$ tsp. garlic powder
Salt and pepper to taste

Directions:
Blend avocados and lemon juice until creamy. Place in a small bowl. Add tomato, onions, and seasonings; mix. Refrigerate until ready to serve.

Saucy Salsa

2 large tomatoes, cored, pureed, and strained
1 large clove garlic, minced
1 chili pepper, coarsely chopped
2 Tbsp. yellow onion, coarsely chopped
$^1/_4$ cup chopped fresh cilantro, rinsed
$^1/_2$ tsp. chopped jalapeno (optional)
2 Tbsp. fresh lemon juice

Directions:
Place tomatoes and garlic in a 2-quart saucepan; boil until tender. Remove from heat; cool. Beat in food processor or with electric mixer until sauce consistency. Add other ingredients; mix. Spoon sauce into a bowl and serve.

Sweet & Sour Sauce

1 (8 oz.) can unsweetened tomato sauce
1 (6 oz.) can tomato paste
1 Tbsp. cold-pressed olive oil
1 tsp. each fresh basil & oregano, chopped
1 tsp. each garlic powder & onion powder
1 $1/4$ cups xylitol

Directions:

Place all ingredients in a large skillet; mix. Bring to a boil, then lower heat. Cover; simmer 20 minutes. Serve over any meat or vegetable dish.

SOUPS

Simply Delicious & Easy Chicken Soup

1 lb. chicken wings
1 (17.5 oz.) can unsweetened chicken broth
3 cups water
1 med. yellow onion, coarsely chopped
1 large carrot, $1/4$-inch rounds
1 stalk celery, diced
$1/4$ tsp. salt
$1/2$ tsp. ground nutmeg

Directions:
Place wings, broth, and water in a 2-quart saucepan; bring to a boil and skim off any foamy substance. Reduce heat; add vegetables and seasonings. Cover; simmer 45 minutes, or until chicken is tender. Remove wings and serve separately or chill and use for chicken salad.

Best Clam Chowder

2 large tomatoes, cored, pureed, and strained
1 cup water
1 (6.5 oz.) can unsweetened minced clams, undrained
2 stalks finely chopped celery
1 med. red bell pepper, diced
1 med. yellow onion, finely chopped
1 large clove garlic, minced
1 Tbsp. each chopped parsley, sage, and thyme
$1/4$ tsp. ground nutmeg

Directions:

Combine all ingredients in a large kettle; mix and bring to a boil. Reduce heat; cover and simmer 15 minutes, or until vegetables are tender.

Black Bean Soup

1 lb. black beans
8 cups vegetable soup stock
1 whole onion
2 bay leaves
1 $\frac{1}{2}$ cups onion, chopped
1 yellow or red pepper, chopped
1 cup celery, chopped (including leaves)
1 cup carrots, grated
1 potato, shredded
2 cloves garlic, minced
Cold-pressed olive oil as needed
2 Tbsp. cilantro
1 tsp. oregano
1 tsp. lemon juice
1 Tbsp. parsley
2 Tbsp. marjoram
1 Tbsp. xylitol
Bragg's Liquid Aminos to taste

Directions:

Sort and rinse black beans; cover with water and soak overnight, then drain. Place beans in a soup pot with vegetable stock, onion, and 2 bay leaves; bring to a boil and cook about 2 $\frac{1}{2}$ hours or until beans are tender. Remove the onion and the bay leaves. Meanwhile combine chopped onion, pepper, celery, carrots, potato, and garlic in a skillet and sauté in a small amount of olive oil until firm but tender. During the last hour of cooking, add the vegetable mixture and seasonings to the beans. Bring to a boil, lower heat to simmer, and cook until vegetables are tender.

Chicken-Egg Drop Soup with Lemon

1 frying chicken (approx. 3 lbs.), quartered
Water
1 med. yellow onion, coarsely chopped
Salt to taste
1 tsp. ground nutmeg
$^1/_2$ cup fresh lemon juice
2 large eggs, beaten
$^1/_4$ tsp. chopped parsley

Directions:
Boil chicken in a large saucepan; reduce heat. Add onion, salt, and nutmeg. Cover and simmer for 1 hour. Remove chicken, reserving broth. Cool. Remove skin and bones; dice chicken meat. Skim any fat off soup, then add chicken and lemon juice. Return broth to heat. Using a teaspoon, drizzle egg into soup.

Chilled Cream of Cucumber Soup

2 $^1/_2$ cups vegetable broth or water
1 Tbsp. Bragg's Liquid Aminos
1 cucumber, peeled & diced
1 onion, chopped
1 cup soft or medium tofu
1 Tbsp. cold-pressed olive oil
Salt & pepper to taste

Directions:

Combine the broth or water, Bragg's Liquid Aminos, cucumber, and onions in a saucepan and bring to a boil. Lower heat, cover and simmer for approximately 15 minutes. Put the tofu, olive oil, and contents from saucepan into a blender and blend thoroughly. Season to taste, let cool, then chill.

Meatball Chowder

1 lb. ground chuck
1 Tbsp. cold-pressed olive oil
6 cups fresh tomatoes, peeled & diced
6 cups pure beef broth
2 cups carrots, thinly sliced
1 medium new potato, diced
1 cup celery, chopped fine
1 Tbsp. fresh parsley
$^1/_2$ tsp. thyme
$^1/_4$ tsp. each basil & garlic powder
2 tsp. salt
$^1/_4$ tsp. pepper

Directions:

Shape ground chuck into meatballs. In large soup pot, brown meatballs in olive oil. When thoroughly browned, add all other ingredients and cook about 1 hour or until tender. Serve immediately.

Meat & Vegetable Soup

1–2 lbs. lean meat, 1-inch cubes
12 cups of water
1 cup carrots, cut in coins
1 cup celery, diced with tops
$^1/_2$ med. green pepper, diced
1 large onion, diced
$^1/_2$ (10 oz.) pkg. frozen green beans
1 cup frozen peas
1 (6 oz.) can tomato paste
2 Tbsp. salt
Sprinkles of garlic powder, pepper, oregano, and dill

Directions:

Combine all ingredients in a large saucepan and bring to a boil. Boil 10 minutes; reduce heat to simmer $2^1/_2$ hours or until meat is tender. Refrigerate overnight. Skim fat from top, then heat and serve.

VEGETABLES AND SIDE DISHES

Shrimp-Stuffed Cherry Tomatoes

$^1/_3$ lb. baby shrimp, cooked
1 stalk celery, finely chopped
$^1/_2$ tsp. garlic powder
$^1/_2$ tsp. chopped fresh basil
2 Tbsp. blender mayonnaise (see page 259)
1 dozen cherry tomatoes, scrubbed & pulp removed
Fresh parsley sprigs for garnish

Directions:

Combine shrimp, celery, garlic powder, basil, and mayonnaise in a small mixing bowl. Place tomatoes on a serving platter; stuff with filling. Place parsley sprigs between and around tomatoes to garnish. Chill 1–2 hours before serving to allow flavors to blend.

Asparagus Sauté

1 lb. fresh asparagus, cut into 2-inch pieces
2 Tbsp. cold-pressed olive oil
Grated fresh gingerroot to taste
2 large cloves garlic, minced

2 Tbsp. sesame seeds
$^1/_4$ tsp. onion powder
$^1/_2$ tsp. salt

Directions:

Place asparagus in a large pot; cover with water. Bring to a boil, reduce heat, and cook 5 minutes; drain. Heat oil in a large skillet. Add ginger, garlic, salt, onion powder, sesame seeds, and asparagus. Sauté, stirring frequently, until tender.

Florentine-Stuffed Tomatoes

$^1/_2$ lb. ground beef
2 Tbsp. cold-pressed olive oil, plus additional for sautéing
1 large clove garlic, minced
1 med. yellow onion, minced
6 large fresh tomatoes
1 (10 oz.) pkg. frozen chopped spinach, thawed & drained
1 Tbsp. fresh basil, coarsely chopped
$^1/_4$ cup ground fresh almonds

Directions:

Preheat oven to 400°F. Brown meat in skillet with olive oil; add garlic and onion; sauté until tender; set aside. Cut tops off tomatoes; remove pulp. Chop pulp; place into a small bowl and reserve. Heat olive oil in another large skillet. Add drained spinach, tomato pulp, and basil. Stir until spinach and tomato are well coated with seasonings; remove from heat. Add meat mixture to spinach. Place tomatoes in a greased 8-inch baking dish; fill with stuffing. Top with almonds. Bake 15–20 minutes.

Japanese Mixed Vegetables & Tofu

$^3/_4$ cup medium tofu
2 Tbsp. cold-pressed olive oil, plus additional for deep-frying
1 small eggplant, thinly sliced
1 onion, thinly sliced
1 clove garlic, crushed
$^1/_2$ cup cabbage
$^1/_2$ cup broccoli
$^1/_2$ cup green beans
1 bell pepper
2 stalks celery
1 (5 oz.) can bamboo shoots
$^2/_3$ cup water
1 tsp. black pepper
2 Tbsp. Bragg's Liquid Aminos
Salt to taste

Directions:

Dice the tofu and deep-fry in olive oil. Drain and set aside. Salt the eggplant slices; set aside with a weight on them for about 30 minutes, then rinse and pat dry. Heat 2 tablespoons olive oil in a wok or large frying pan and sauté onion and garlic until lightly browned. Chop the cabbage coarsely. Cut the broccoli into florets. Slice the beans, bell pepper, and celery. Add these vegetables, the eggplant, and bamboo shoots to the onion and garlic. Stir-fry for 3–5 minutes. Add water, black pepper, Bragg's Liquid Aminos and salt; bring to a boil, then reduce heat and simmer for 5–10 minutes. Add the tofu and simmer for another 5–10 minutes before serving.

Chicken Salad

3 cups chicken, deboned
1 stalk celery, chopped
$^1/_4$ cup cucumber, chopped
$^1/_3$ cup onion, diced
$^1/_4$ cup blender mayonnaise (see page 259)
1 tsp. mild mustard (see page 260)

Directions:

Boil chicken. Combine vegetables, mayonnaise, and mustard in a large serving bowl. Season mixture to taste. Place in refrigerator to cool for several hours. Serve on crisp lettuce leaves. (Chicken may easily be substituted with tuna, turkey, or ham if desired.)

Scrumptious Zucchini Sauté

2 Tbsp. cold-pressed olive oil
1 lb. zucchini, shredded
1 large tomato, coarsely chopped
3 small green onions, coarsely chopped
2 large cloves garlic, minced
Coarsely chopped fresh basil to taste
$^1/_4$ tsp. thyme
Salt to taste

Directions:

Heat oil in a large nonstick skillet. Add garlic; sauté 2–3 minutes until tender. Add all other ingredients; sauté, stirring frequently, 2–3 minutes until cooked but not overdone.

Fancy Red & Green Slaw

1 green cabbage, grated
1 red cabbage, grated
3 green onions
$^1/_4$ cup blender mayonnaise (see page 259)
$^1/_4$ cup xylitol
2 tsp. caraway seeds
Salt to taste

Directions:

Mix all ingredients in a large bowl. Refrigerate at least 1 hour before serving to allow flavors to blend.

Tofu & Vegetable Salad

2 cups firm tofu
3 spring onions (scallions), chopped
1 green bell pepper, chopped
2 stalks celery, chopped
1 carrot, grated
6 Tbsp. blender mayonnaise (see page 259)

Directions:

Cut tofu into small cubes. Combine vegetables and tofu in a bowl and stir in the mayonnaise. Chill before serving.

MAIN DISHES

Chili Con Tofu

1 cup fresh tofu
2 onions, finely chopped
2 Tbsp. cold-pressed olive oil
1 carrot, chopped
1 stalk celery, finely chopped
1 small bell pepper, finely chopped
1 clove garlic, finely chopped
4 small tomatoes, finely chopped
1 lb. drained cooked kidney beans
2 Tbsp. water
2 tsp. Bragg's Liquid Aminos
2 Tbsp. tomato paste
2 tsp. Mexican chili seasoning

Directions:

Drain tofu thoroughly and squeeze the moisture out. Set aside. Sauté onions in olive oil for 3–4 minutes over low heat until just tender. Add carrots, celery, and green bell pepper to the onions. Stir well and cool for 2–3 minutes. Add garlic to saucepan, stir well, and cook for an additional 4–5 minutes. Add tomatoes, kidney beans, water, Bragg's Liquid Aminos, tomato paste, and chili seasoning to the pan. Crumble the tofu into the saucepan. Stir well. Cover the saucepan and leave to simmer over low heat for 10–15 minutes, stirring occasionally. Serve immediately.

Mexican Omelets

2 $2/3$ tsp. cold-pressed olive oil, divided

2 cups onion, minced

4 garlic cloves, minced, divided

$1/2$ cup cooked garbanzo beans

$1/2$ cup cooked kidney beans

1 cup red bell pepper, diced

1 cup green bell pepper, diced

2 whole eggs

12 egg whites

$1/8$ tsp. dry mustard

$1/4$ tsp. turmeric

$1/8$ tsp. chili powder

$1/8$ tsp. black pepper

Cayenne pepper to taste

Directions:

In a medium nonstick sauté pan, cook onion, garlic, garbanzo beans, kidney beans, and red and green peppers in $2/3$ teaspoon olive oil until tender. In a mixing bowl, whip together whole eggs, egg whites, mustard, turmeric, chili powder, black pepper, and cayenne pepper. In a second sauté pan, heat 1 teaspoon olive oil before adding half the egg mixture. Cook until set and an omelet is formed. Fill omelet with half the vegetable mixture; fold over and serve. Repeat process to make second omelet.

Scrambled Eggs with a Flair

8 large eggs
$^1/_2$ lb. cooked baby shrimp, rinsed
1 med. avocado, peeled & diced
1 med. red bell pepper, diced
2 med. green onions, diced
$^1/_2$ tsp. garlic powder
Cayenne pepper to taste
2 Tbsp. cold-pressed olive oil

Directions:
Beat eggs in a large bowl. Add rest of ingredients, except olive oil; mix. Heat olive oil in large nonstick skillet; add egg mixture. Cook over medium-high heat, stirring frequently, until eggs are set. Serve immediately.

Hamburger in a Skillet

1 lb. ground beef
$^1/_2$ cup diced onion
2 cups beef broth
$1^1/_2$ cups water
$^1/_4$ tsp. garlic salt
1 (10 oz.) pkg. frozen peas, thawed
1 (5 oz.) can water chestnuts

Directions:
In a large skillet, brown meat and onion; pour off grease. Add broth, water, and garlic salt to skillet. Reduce heat to low; simmer 15 minutes. Stir in peas and water chestnuts. Heat through; serve.

Tofu Rancheros

1 onion, chopped
1 green bell pepper, chopped
1 red bell pepper, chopped
2 Tbsp. cold-pressed olive oil
2 Tbsp. Mexican chili seasoning
$1/2$ tsp. turmeric
$1/4$ cup soy flour
1 (14–16 oz.) can tomatoes, drained
2 cups firm tofu

Directions:

Sauté onion and bell peppers in olive oil until tender. Add the chili seasoning, turmeric, and soy flour. Stir well, then slowly add the tomatoes. Bring to a boil, lower heat, and simmer for about 5 minutes. Place tofu on a clean towel and squeeze well to extract moisture. Crumble tofu, then add to tomato mixture. Heat for 1–2 minutes before serving.

Crockpot Chicken

1 whole chicken (approx. $2\,1/2$–3 lbs.)
$2/3$ cup onions, chopped
$1/2$ cup celery, chopped
$1/2$ cup carrots, sliced
Salt & pepper to taste

Directions:

Place chicken in crockpot. Add 2–3 cups water along with onion, celery, and carrots. Sprinkle with salt and pepper. Cook on low for 4–6 hours. When tender, remove skin and serve.

Pepper Steak

2 lbs. round steak, cut into thin strips
$^1/_3$ cup cold-pressed olive oil
1 tsp. salt
Dash pepper
Dash garlic powder
$^1/_4$ cup Bragg's Liquid Aminos
1 sliced green pepper
1 can bean sprouts, drained
1 onion, chopped
2 tomatoes, quartered
1 Tbsp. potato starch

Directions:

Brown meat in olive oil in large frying pan. Add seasonings and stir occasionally. Cover and cook over low heat 30 minutes or until tender. Add Bragg's Liquid Aminos, green pepper, bean sprouts, and onion. Cover and cook another 5 minutes. Add tomatoes. Blend potato starch with water and add to meat mixture. Cook, stirring gently, until sauce is thick.

Roasted Herb Chicken

1 whole roasting chicken (approx. 3 lbs.)
Cold-pressed olive oil
Salt to taste
Chopped fresh rosemary & tarragon to taste
2 Tbsp. soy flour
$^1/_2$ cup unsweetened chicken broth

Directions:

Preheat oven to 350°F. Place chicken in a large baking dish or roasting pan. Rub olive oil over chicken; sprinkle seasonings over top and sides. Cover dish or pan with foil; bake 45 minutes, basting frequently. Remove foil; bake 15–20 minutes, or until browned. Remove from oven. Pour drippings into a 2-quart saucepan. Mix flour and broth in a measuring cup; pour into saucepan and stir until gravy thickens. Simmer 5 minutes. Cut chicken into pieces. Serve the gravy over the chicken, or on the side.

Beef Burgers

$1^1/_2$ lbs. ground beef
$^3/_4$ cup rolled oats
$^1/_2$ cup onion, chopped
$^1/_3$ cup tomato puree
1 egg
1 tsp. salt
$^1/_8$ tsp. pepper

Directions:

Combine all ingredients; mix well. Shape to form six 3-inch patties. Cook in broiler or grill 5–6 minutes per side or until desired doneness.

Grandma's Chili

1 Tbsp. cold-pressed olive oil
1 lb. ground chuck
1 onion, chopped
1 green bell pepper, chopped
3 cloves garlic, minced
1 (14–16 oz.) can red beans, drained
1 (14–16 oz.) can chopped tomatoes with juice
1 (6 oz.) can tomato paste
2 tsp. chili powder
1 tsp. ground cumin
1 tsp. salt
Water or vegetable broth if needed

Directions:
Heat olive oil in a 2-quart saucepan; brown meat, onion, bell pepper, and garlic. Add remaining ingredients. Bring to a boil, then reduce heat to simmer. Cook covered 1 hour, stirring occasionally to avoid burning.

Tuna-Almond Casserole

$1/2$ cup onion, chopped
$1/2$ green pepper, chopped
$1/2$ cup slivered almonds, divided
$1/4$ cup cold-pressed olive oil
1 (8 oz.) can water-packed tuna, drained

Directions:
Preheat oven to 425°F. In a large skillet, lightly sauté onion, bell pepper, and $1/4$ cup almonds in olive oil. Combine with tuna. Put in casserole dish; cover with remaining almonds. Bake 15 minutes.

Filet of Sole

4 filets of sole (6–8 oz. each)
$^{1}/_{2}$ cup cold-pressed olive oil
1 tsp. garlic powder
$^{1}/_{2}$ tsp. each chopped fresh basil & oregano
Salt, pepper, and paprika to taste
2 oz. slivered almonds

Directions:

Preheat oven to 350°F. Arrange filets in a shallow baking dish. Brush lightly with olive oil; sprinkle with seasonings. Bake uncovered for 20 minutes. Remove from oven and sprinkle with almond slivers, then bake for another 10–15 minutes longer if necessary, or until fork-tender.

Stuffed Salmon for Two

2 Tbsp. cold-pressed olive oil
$^1/_4$ lb. cooked baby shrimp, chopped
$^1/_4$ lb. crab meat
$^1/_2$ med. yellow onion, finely chopped
$^1/_2$ med. lemon, peeled & finely chopped
1 Tbsp. fresh parsley, finely chopped
$^1/_2$ Tbsp. fresh dill weed, chopped
$^1/_2$ tsp. garlic powder
$^1/_4$ tsp. salt
2 salmon filets (6–8 oz. each)

Directions:

Preheat oven to 350°F. Heat olive oil in a small skillet; add shrimp, crab meat, onion, lemon, and remaining seasonings; mix and remove from heat. Cut filets into halves. Place one half filet (skin side down) in the center of a 12-inch piece of foil. Repeat, using the other half filet and placing on a second sheet of foil. Spread shrimp and crab mixture over filets on foil; top with other filet halves (skin side up). Secure with toothpicks. Fold foil over filets; seal. Place in an 8-inch baking dish; bake 25 minutes.

Veal with Italian Vegetables

$2\,^2/_3$ tsp. cold-pressed olive oil, divided

3 cups eggplant, $^1/_2$-inch cubes

3 cups zucchini, $^1/_2$-inch cubes

2 cups tomato, $^1/_2$-inch cubes

1 cup onion rings, halved

4 garlic cloves, minced

$^1/_2$ tsp. dried marjoram

$^1/_8$ tsp. dried sage

$^1/_2$ tsp. dried oregano

$^1/_2$ cup tomato puree

6 oz. veal scaloppini

2 Tbsp. water

$^1/_8$ tsp. dried rosemary

$^1/_8$ tsp. onion powder

2 Tbsp.+ $^1/_8$ tsp. dried basil

$^1/_8$ tsp. salt

$^1/_8$ tsp. pepper

Directions:

Heat 2 tablespoons olive oil in a sauté pan. Sauté vegetables, garlic, marjoram, sage, and oregano. Cook until almost tender, then add tomato puree. While the vegetables are continuing to cook, place veal in a second sauté pan with $^2/_3$ teaspoon olive oil and 2 tablespoons water. Cook veal until browned; sprinkle with rosemary, onion powder, basil, salt, and pepper. Divide veal and vegetables; serve.

Pork Meatballs with Tomato-Tarragon Sauce

12 oz. lean ground pork
1 cup lentils, cooked
1 cup onion, diced
$1/4$ tsp. chili powder
$1/8$ tsp. dried basil
$1/8$ tsp. dried tarragon, divided
$1/8$ tsp. black pepper
$1/8$ tsp. dried marjoram, divided
$2\,2/3$ tsp. cold-pressed olive oil
1 cup tomato puree
$1/2$ cup beef broth
2 tsp. lemon juice

Directions:

Preheat oven to 375°F. In a large mixing bowl, combine pork, lentils, onion, chili powder, basil, a dash of tarragon, pepper, and a dash of marjoram. Form mixture into 16 one-inch meatballs. Place meatballs in a baking dish brushed with olive oil; bake for 15 minutes. Meanwhile, in a small saucepan, combine tomato puree, beef broth, lemon juice, a dash of tarragon, and a dash of marjoram. Simmer 3–4 minutes to heat through. Remove meatballs from oven and gently place in sauce.; spoon rest of sauce over meatballs. Serve.

Chicken Cacciatore

1 frying chicken (approximately 3 lbs.), quartered
Garlic powder to taste
$^1/_2$ onion, chopped
Fresh basil to taste
1 (8 oz.) can unsweetened tomato sauce
$^3/_4$ tsp. Italian seasoning

Directions:

Preheat oven to 375°F. Place chicken quarters, skin side up, in a greased baking dish. Sprinkle seasonings and onions over top. Bake 30 minutes; turn and season other side. Bake 20 minutes longer. Spoon $^1/_2$ can tomato sauce over chicken parts. Sprinkle more seasonings over sauce; spoon rest of sauce over top. Season and bake 10–15 minutes or until tender.

Greek Shish Kebab

1 $^1/_2$ lb. round steak cut into 1-inch cubes
$^1/_2$ cup cold-pressed olive oil
3 Tbsp. lemon concentrate
$^1/_4$ tsp. oregano
2 Tbsp. carrots, finely chopped
2 Tbsp. celery, finely chopped
Vegetable squares of your choice

Directions:

Combine all ingredients and leave meat to marinate approximately 3 hours. Thread onto skewers with vegetable squares of your choice. Cook under broiler or grill until done.

Tangy Chicken & Bean Salad

$2\,^2/_3$ tsp. cold-pressed olive oil

8 oz. chicken tenderloins (or skinless chicken breast), cubed

1 cup fresh green beans, $^1/_2$" pieces

$^1/_4$ cup kidney beans, cooked

1 cup onion, diced

$^1/_4$ cup garbanzo beans, rinsed

$^1/_4$ cup water

$^1/_4$ cup lemon juice

$^1/_4$ tsp. celery salt

$^1/_8$ tsp. dry mustard

$^1/_8$ tsp. cayenne pepper

$^1/_8$ tsp. chili powder

$^1/_8$ tsp. curry powder

$^1/_2$ head lettuce, shredded

6 cups spinach

$1\,^1/_4$ cups tomato, diced

1 cucumber, peeled & diced

Directions:

In medium sauté pan, add 2 teaspoons olive oil, chicken, green beans, kidney beans, onion, and garbanzo beans. Cook on medium-high heat for 10–15 minutes until the chicken is done and vegetables are crispy-tender. While the chicken and vegetables are cooking, heat $^2/_3$ teaspoon olive oil, water, lemon juice, and spices in a medium saucepan. Bring to a boil, then add to the chicken and vegetable mixture; stir.

In a large salad bowl, combine the lettuce, spinach, tomato, and cucumber to form a salad. Top the salad with the chicken mixture and serve.

Curried Lamb Stew

4 Tbsp. cold-pressed olive oil
1 lb. lamb shoulder, cut into bite-size pieces
$^1/_4$ cup potato flour
1 med. yellow onion, chopped
2 med. new potatoes, peeled & diced
2 tsp. curry powder
1 tsp. garlic powder
$^1/_2$ tsp. salt
1 (10 oz.) pkg. frozen peas, thawed

Directions:
Preheat oven to 375°F. Heat olive oil in a large skillet. Coat lamb with potato flour. Add to skillet, then add onion, potatoes, and seasonings. Sauté over medium-high heat until lightly browned, turning often. Add peas; stir mixture and remove from heat. Spoon into an 8-inch greased casserole dish. Bake 1 hour.

Lemon Pepper Chicken

4 skinless chicken breast halves
Lemon pepper to taste
1 lemon, cut in 8 slices
Parsley

Directions:
Place chicken in 8x8 greased baking dish. Preheat oven to 350°F (325°F if using a glass baking dish). Sprinkle chicken lightly with lemon pepper. Place 2 lemon slices on each chicken breast. Sprinkle with parsley. Bake for 45–60 minutes or until chicken is cooked through and tender.

Baked Italian Trout

2 trout filets
Black olives
Cayenne pepper to taste
Salt & pepper to taste
1 small lemon, peeled & thinly sliced
$^1/_2$ yellow onion, thinly sliced
1 can Italian stewed tomatoes

Directions:
Place filets in small greased baking dish. Season filets to taste. Cover filets with lemon, onion, tomatoes, and olives. Bake at 350°F until lightly brown.

Baked Lemon Turkey Breast

$^1/_2$ turkey breast (about 3–4 lbs.)
$^1/_2$ can unsweetened chicken broth
1 large clove garlic, minced
1 med. lemon, sliced into rounds
1 med. yellow onion, sliced
Chopped fresh sage & basil to taste
Salt to taste
Parsley sprigs for garnish

Directions:
Preheat oven to 325°F. Place turkey in a large baking dish; cover with broth. Cut several slits in top of breast skin; plug with garlic. Place lemon slices on top of turkey; surround bottom of breast with onion. Sprinkle seasonings over breast; bake 20 minutes per pound, basting as needed. When browned, cover pan with foil; then bake 30–50 minutes. Let sit a few minutes before slicing.

Mama's Meat Loaf

2 lbs. ground chuck
1 (10 oz.) can tomato paste
1 egg
1 onion, grated
1 bell pepper, chopped
1 clove garlic, minced
$^3/_4$ cup rolled oats
1 $^1/_2$ tsp. salt
$^1/_4$ tsp. pepper
1 (6 oz.) can tomato paste, for sauce

Directions:

Combine all ingredients except 6 oz. can tomato paste in large bowl, mixing well. Place in loaf pan; using knife, poke holes in loaf. Pour the 6 oz. can of tomato paste over top of loaf, then bake at 350°F for 1 $^1/_2$ hours.

Shrimp Curry

$^1/_2$ cup onion, finely chopped
1 $^1/_2$ Tbsp. cold-pressed olive oil
2 Tbsp. potato starch
1 tsp. seasoned salt
1 tsp. curry powder
$^1/_4$ tsp. pepper
2 cups pure chicken broth
2 cups fresh shrimp, cooked

Directions:

Sauté onions in olive oil for 5 minutes. Blend in potato starch and seasonings. Slowly add broth, stirring constantly. Bring to a boil; reduce heat and simmer gently about 10 minutes, stirring occasionally. Add shrimp and heat through.

Chicken Stir-Fry

2 whole chicken breasts, deboned
2 Tbsp. cold-pressed olive oil
1 med. green bell pepper, cut into strips
1 med. yellow bell pepper, cut into strips
1 small onion, thinly sliced
1 cup celery, thinly sliced
1 (5 oz.) can water chestnuts, drained & sliced
$^1/_2$ cup water
2 cloves garlic, chopped
$^1/_2$ tsp. ground ginger
Salt & pepper to taste
4 tsp. potato starch
4 Tbsp. pure chicken broth
1 (16 oz.) can bean sprouts

Directions:

Remove skin and cut chicken into thin strips. Heat olive oil in a large skillet; add chicken and cook over medium heat 4 or 5 minutes or until meat turns white. Add bell peppers, onion, celery, water chestnuts, water, garlic, ginger, salt, and pepper. Cover and cook over medium-low heat, approximately 5 minutes. Blend potato starch and broth together; stir into chicken mixture. Add bean sprouts and cook about 2 minutes more or until thickened, stirring constantly.

Mulligan Stew

1 lb. beef, cut into small pieces

1 Tbsp. cold-pressed olive oil

1 tsp. salt

1 (10 oz.) can tomato puree

2 cups water

3 carrots sliced

1 med. new potato, chopped

2 onions, each cut into 4 pieces

Directions:

In a skillet, brown beef with olive oil over medium heat. Add salt, tomato puree, and water; cover tightly; cook slowly until tender. Add carrots, potatoes, and onions; cover and continue cooking about 30 minutes. Add water, if needed. If stew is too thin, remove lid and cook until thickened.

Sweet & Sour Pork & Cabbage

8 oz. pork loin
Salt and pepper to taste
$2^2/_3$ tsp. cold-pressed olive oil
6 cups cabbage, shredded
1 cup garbanzo beans, chopped
1 cup water chestnuts
2 cups celery, chopped
1 cup bok choy
1 cup bamboo shoots
10 Tbsp. lemon juice
$^1/_2$ cup water

Directions:

Cut the pork tenderloin into $^1/_2$-inch cubes; salt and pepper pork to taste. Brown pork with $^2/_3$ tsp. olive oil in a nonstick sauté pan. Set aside. Add cabbage, garbanzo beans, water chestnuts, celery, bok choy, bamboo shoots, lemon juice, and 2 teaspoons olive oil to sauté pan and cook vegetable mixture for 10–15 minutes, until vegetables are almost tender. Add water and cooked pork to vegetables; cover. Braise mixture for 5–10 minutes, stirring occasionally.

Stuffed Pork with Cashews & Vegetable Sauce

Pork chops:
$2^2/_3$ tsp. cold-pressed olive oil
$^1/_2$ cup cooked snow peas, chopped
$^1/_8$ tsp. Bragg's Liquid Aminos
$^1/_8$ tsp. black pepper
$^1/_8$ tsp. marjoram
$^1/_2$ cup onion, diced
2 boneless pork chops (4 oz. each)

Sauce:
3 cups chicken broth
2 cups celery, chopped
$1^1/_2$ cups broccoli, chopped
2 cups cauliflower, chopped
$2^1/_4$ cups red bell pepper, diced
$^1/_8$ tsp. basil
$^1/_8$ tsp. cinnamon & nutmeg
$^1/_2$ cup cashew nuts
Salt to taste
4 tsp. cornstarch

Directions:

Pork chops: Preheat oven to 375°F. In a sauté pan, add $^2/_3$ tsp. olive oil, snow peas, Bragg's Liquid Aminos, black pepper, marjoram, and onions. Cook until mixture is translucent (about 10 minutes). Set aside to cool. Slice pork chops and fill with mixture; secure with toothpicks. Bake at 375°F for 20–25 minutes in a covered baking dish.

Sauce: While the pork chops are cooking, combine chicken broth, celery, broccoli, cauliflower, bell pepper, basil, cinnamon, and nutmeg in a saucepan. Bring to a boil and cook until vegetables are tender. Reduce heat, add cashews, and simmer for 5 minutes; add salt to taste. Combine cornstarch with water to form smooth paste and add to mixture until a sauce forms.

Appendix F
A Simple At-Home Test of Thyroid Function

A safe, easy way to evaluate your thyroid function at home is by measuring your basal body temperature, your body's core temperature when you are completely at rest. Because heat is a measure of energy, your basal body temperature reflects your body's energy production and metabolic rate, which in turn reflects your thyroid function.

To measure your basal body temperature, place a thermometer beside your bed when you go to sleep. Upon waking, place the thermometer under your arm and lie completely still for ten minutes. Then record the temperature. Repeat this procedure every morning for five days. To determine your average basal body temperature, add the temperature readings for these five days and divide the total by five.

Men and non-menstruating females can perform this test at any time during the month. Because basal body temperature fluctuates during the menstrual cycle, women who are menstruating should begin measuring their temperature on the second day of their menstrual period and continue for five days.

A normal basal body temperature is between 97.8 and 98.2 degrees. If your average basal body temperature over a five-day period is below 97.8, then it is likely that you have hypothyroidism.

APPENDIX G
Resources

WELLNESS MEDICINE

Hotze Health & Wellness Center
877-698-8698 or 281-579-3600
www.hotzehwc.com

American Academy of Biologically
Identical Hormone Therapy
281-828-0026
www.aabiht.com

BIOIDENTICAL HORMONES SPECIALTY PHARMACY

Premier Pharmacy
877-640-5248 or 281-829-9088
www.premier-pharmacy.com

Vitamins and Nutritional Supplements

Physician's Preference ®
800-579-6545 or 281-646-1659
www.physicianspreference.com

Bioidentical Hormone Treatment Information

Hotze Health & Wellness Center
877-698-8698 or 281-579-3600
www.hotzehwc.com

John R. Lee, M.D.
www.johnleemd.com

Thyroid Information

Broda O. Barnes, M.D., Research Foundation, Inc.
www.brodabarnes.org

ALLERGY INFORMATION

Hotze Health & Wellness Center
877-698-8698 or 281-579-3600
www.hotzehwc.com

Pan American Allergy Society
www.paas.org

American Academy of Otolaryngic Allergy
www.aaoaf.org

Allergy Choices
www.allergychoices.com

YEAST (CANDIDA) INFORMATION

Hotze Health & Wellness Center
877-698-8698 or 281-579-3600
www.hotzehwc.com

The Yeast Connection
www.yeastconnection.com

HEALTH & WELLNESS SOLUTIONS RADIO PROGRAM

In Houston, 700 AM KSEV, Monday through Thursday, noon to 1 p.m.

www.ksevradio.com

APPENDIX H
Bibliography

BOOKS

The information in this book is based on research published in medical journals and textbooks and the clinical experience of the physicians at the Hotze Health & Wellness Center. If you would like to learn more about the topics presented in this book, I recommend consulting the following texts, which are written for lay readers.

Barnes, Broda O., M.D, and Lawrence Galton. *Hypothyroidism: The Unsuspected Illness.* New York: Harper & Row, 1976.

Brownstein, David, M.D. *The Miracle of Natural Hormones.* West Bloomfield, MI: Medical Alternatives Press, 2003.

Crook, William G., M.D. *The Yeast Connection.* New York: Vintage Books, 1983.

Diamond, Jed. *Male Menopause.* Naperville, IL: Sourcebooks, 1998.

Ford, Gillian. *Listening to Your Hormones.* Rocklin, CA: Prima Lifestyles, 1997.

Graedon, Joe, and Teresa Graedon, Ph.D. *Deadly Drug Interactions*. New York: St. Martin's Press, 1995.

Hufnagel, Vicki, M.D., with Susan K. Golant. *No More Hysterectomies*. New York: Penguin Books, 1989.

Jefferies, William McK., M.D. *Safe Uses of Cortisol.* Springfield, IL: Charles C. Thomas, 1996.

Lee, John R., M.D., et al. *What Your Doctor May Not Tell You About Breast Cancer.* New York: Warner Books, 2003.

Lee, John R., M.D., et al. *What Your Doctor May Not Tell You About Premenopause.* New York: Warner Books, 1999.

Lee, John R., M.D., with Virginia Hopkins. *What Your Doctor May Not Tell You About Menopause.* New York: Warner Books, 1996.

Mendelsohn, Robert S., M.D. *Confessions of a Medical Heretic.* Lincolnwood, IL: Contemporary Books, 1979.

Mindell, Earl. *Earl Mindell's Vitamin Bible.* New York: Warner Books, 1991.

Nuland, Sherwin B. *The Doctors' Plague.* New York: Atlas Books, 2003.

Reiss, Uzzi, M.D., with Martin Zucker. *Natural Hormone Balance for Women.* New York: Atria Books, 2002.

Sears, Barry, Ph.D., with Bill Lawren. *Enter the Zone*. New York: Regan Books, 1995.

Sears, Barry, Ph.D., with Mary Goodbody. *Mastering the Zone*. New York: Regan Books, 1996.

Sears, Barry, Ph.D. *The Anti-Aging Zone*. New York: Regan Books, 1999.

Shippen, Eugene, M.D., and William Fryer. *The Testosterone Syndrome*. New York: M. Evans & Co., 2001.

Szasz, Thomas S., M.D. *The Myth of Mental Illness*. New York: Harper & Row, 1974.

Whitaker, Julian M., M.D. *Dr. Whitaker's Guide to Natural Hormone Replacement*. Potomac, MD: Phillips Publishing, 1998.

Whitaker, Julian M., M.D. *Reversing Heart Disease*. New York: Warner Books, 2002.

JOURNALS

The journal articles below contain key studies pertaining to bioidentical hormones, nutritional supplements, allergy treatment, and other topics discussed in this book. Abstracts of most of these studies can be found on PubMed, a service of the National Library of Medicine, located at http://www.ncbi.nlm .nih.gov/entrez/query.fcgi?db=PubMed.

Age-Related Eye Disease Study Research Group. A randomized, placebo-controlled, clinical trial of high-dose supplementation with vitamins C and E, beta carotene, and zinc for age-related macular degeneration and vision loss: AREDS report no. 8. *Arch Ophthalmol* 2001;119:1417–36.

Bera, V.; Million Women Study Collaborators. Breast cancer and hormone-replacement therapy in the Million Women Study. *Lancet* 2003;362:419–27.

Buck, D. S., et al. Comparison of two topical preparations for the treatment of onychomycosis: *Melaleuca alternifolia* (tea tree) oil and clotrimazole. *J Fam Pract* 1994;38:601–5.

Bunevicius, R., et al. Effects of thyroxine as compared with thyroxine plus triiodothyronine in patients with hypothyroidism. *N Engl J Med* 1999;340:424–9.

Clark, L. C., et al. Effects of selenium supplementation for cancer prevention in patients with carcinoma of the skin. *JAMA* 1996;276:1957–63.

Coronary artery surgery study (CASS): a randomized trial of coronary artery bypass surgery. Survival data. *Circulation* 1983;68:939–950.

Cowan, L. D., et al. Breast cancer incidence in women with a history of progesterone deficiency. *Am J Epidemiol* 1981;114:209–17.

de Lignieres, B. Oral micronized progesterone. *Clin Therapeutics* 1999;21:41–60.

Ervin, R. B., and J. Kennedy-Stephenson. Mineral intakes of elderly adult supplement and non-supplement users in the Third National Health and Nutrition Examination Survey. *J Nutr* 2002;132:3422–7.

Graham, I. M., et al. Plasma homocysteine as a risk factor for vascular disease. *JAMA* 1997;277:1775–81.

Laumann, E. O., et al. Sexual dysfunction in the United States: Prevalence and predictors. *JAMA* 1999;281:537–44.

McCaig L. F., and J. M. Hughes. Trends in antimicrobial drug prescribing among office-based physicians in the United States. *JAMA* 1995;273:214–9.

McCullough, M. L., et al. Calcium, vitamin D, dairy products, and risk of colorectal cancer in the Cancer Prevention Study II Nutrition Cohort. *Cancer Causes Control* 2003;14:1–12.

Ponikau, J. U., et al. The diagnosis and incidence of allergic fungal sinusitis. *Mayo Clin Proc* 1999;74:877–84.

Rimm, E. B., et al. Folate and vitamin B_6 from diet and supplements in relation to risk of coronary heart disease among women. *JAMA* 1998;279:359–64.

Rossouw, J. E., et al. Risks and benefits of estrogen plus progestin in healthy postmenopausal women: Principle results from the Women's Health Initiative randomized controlled trial. *JAMA* 2002;288:321–33.

Shumaker, S. A., et al. Estrogen plus progestin and the incidence of dementia and mild cognitive impairment in postmenopausal women: The Women's Health Initiative Memory Study: a randomized controlled trial. *JAMA* 2003;289:2651–62.

Stampfer, M. J., et al. A prospective study of plasma homocyst(e) ine and risk of myocardial infarction in U.S. physicians. *JAMA* 1992;268:877–81.

Stephens, N. G., et al. Randomised controlled trial of vitamin E in patients with coronary disease: Cambridge Heart Antioxidant Study (CHAOS). *Lancet* 1996;347:781–6.

Thomas, M. K., et al. Hypovitaminosis D in medical inpatients. *N Engl J Med* 1998;338:777–83.

Tice, J. A., et al. Cost-effectiveness of vitamin therapy to lower plasma homocysteine levels for the prevention of coronary heart disease: Effect of grain fortification and beyond. *JAMA* 2001;286:936–43.

Tucker, K. L., et al. Plasma vitamin B-12 concentrations relate to intake source in the Framingham Offspring study. *Am J Clin Nutr* 2000;71:514–22.

Appendix I
Clinical Studies at the Hotze Health & Wellness Center

I. LONG-TERM TREATMENT OF ALLERGY PATIENTS WITH AUTOIMMUNE THYROIDITIS AT THE HOTZE HEALTH & WELLNESS CENTER

INTRODUCTION

This study was conducted from April 2, 1992 to September 6, 1996, at the Hotze Health & Wellness Center to determine the incidence of autoimmune thyroiditis and low thyroid function (hypothyroidism) among allergy patients and to evaluate the health improvement in these patients when treated with natural thyroid supplementation.

This clinical study was presented by Steven F. Hotze, M.D., at the American Academy of Otolaryngic Allergy Annual Meeting, September 27, 1996, in Washington, D.C., and received the Sanders Award for the best clinical study of the year.

At the Hotze Health & Wellness Center, symptoms of hypothyroidism are treated using Armour Thyroid. The average dose is 2.5 grains per day.

ELECTRONIC MEDIA

Http://www.pbs.org/wgbh/pages/frontline/shows/prescription /interviews/elashoff.html. Date of interview Feb. 19, 2003 (accessed December 31, 2004).

Patient Population

Total number of patients evaluated: 697
Total number of patients with anti-thyroid antibodies ATA: 164

Number of female patients: 407 (58%)
Number of female patients with ATA: 112
(28% of all female patients; 68% of all patients with ATA)

Number of male patients: 290 (42%)
Number of male patients with ATA: 52
(18% of all male patients; 32% of all patients with ATA)
Total number of ATA patients responding to questionnaire
about symptoms: 119
Number of respondents receiving Armour Thyroid: 59 (50%)
Number of female respondents receiving Armour Thyroid:
46 (78%)
Number of male respondents receiving Armour Thyroid:
13 (22%)

Results

The following chart summarizes the improvement in symptoms among patients receiving Armour Thyroid. The average duration of treatment was 3.3 years for female patients and 2.3 years for male patients, and the average dosage of Armour Thyroid was 2.5 grains per day. Not all patients had all symptoms; the statistics represent the percentage improvement among patients who initially reported the symptom.

Percentage of Improvement and/or Resolution of Symptoms of Patients in Study Receiving Armour Thyroid

Symptom	No. of Patients	Symptoms Resolved	Symptoms Improved	Symptoms Unchanged	Worsening of Symptoms
Low Energy	58	0(0%)	50(86%)	8(14%)	0(0%)
Weight Problems	48	0(0%)	21(44%)	17(35%)	10(21%)
Cold Sensitivity	41	20(49%)	13(31%)	4(10%)	4(10%)
Mental Dysfunction	37	8(22%)	14(38%)	15(40%)	0(0%)
Dry Skin	34	2(6%)	11(32%)	10(30%)	11(32%)
Hair Loss	25	11(44%)	5(20%)	7(28%)	2(8%)
Depressed Mood	30	6(20%)	14(47%)	10(33%)	0(0%)
Constipation	17	3(18%)	8(47%)	6(35%)	0(0%)
Fluid Retention	22	6(27%)	9(41%)	4(18%)	3(14%)
Joint Pain	24	4(17%)	8(33%)	8(33%)	4(17%)
Muscle Pain	21	5(24%)	4(19%)	10(47%)	2(10%)
Sleep Disturbance	46	6(13%)	24(51%)	13(28%)	3(6%)

Follow-up Study: Incidence of Autoimmune Thyroiditis in Allergy Patients

An analysis of data from 1,340 patients evaluated between the dates of April 2, 1992, and March 31, 1998, revealed that:
342 patients (25.5%) had anti-thyroid antibodies
255 (75%) of these patients were females
87 (25%) of these patients were males

834 female allergy patients were evaluated during this period
255 (31%) of these female patients had anti-thyroid antibodies
506 male allergy patients were evaluated during this period
87 (17%) of these male patients had anti-thyroid antibodies

Conclusion

This study shows that autoimmune thyroiditis and symptoms of hypothyroidism are very common among allergy patients, especially female allergy patients. When indicated, natural thyroid supplementation using Armour Thyroid benefits these patients by relieving their hypothyroid symptoms, thus improving their overall health and sense of well-being.

REFERENCES

Dayan, C. M., and D. H. Daniels. Chronic autoimmune thyroiditis. *N Engl J Med* 1996;335:99–107.

DeRosa, G., et al. A slightly suppressive dose of L-thyroxine does not affect bone turnover and bone mineral density in pre- and postmenopausal women with nontoxic goiter. *Horm Metab Res* 1995;27:503–7.

Fisher, D., and G. N. Beall. Hashimoto's thyroiditis. *Pharmacological Therapy* 1976;C1:445–8.

Giani, C., et al. Relationship between breast cancer and thyroid disease: Relevance of autoimmune thyroid disorders in breast malignancy. *J Clin Endocrinol Metab* 1996;81:990–4.

Kutty, K. M., et al. Serum lipids in hypothyroidism a re-evaluation. *J Clin Endocrinol Metab* 1978;46:55–6.

Phillips, D., et al. Autosomal dominant inheritance of autoantibodies to thyroid peroxidase and thyroglobulin studies in families not selected for autoimmune thyroid disease. *J Clin Endocrinol Metab* 1991;72:973–5.

Phillips, D., et al. Autosomal dominant transmission of autoantibodies to thyroglobulin and thyroid peroxidase. *J Clin Endocrinol Metab* 1990;70:742–6.

Rumbyrt, J. S., et al. Resolution of chronic urticaria in patients with thyroid autoimmunity. *J Allergy Clin Immuno* 1995;96:901–5.

Stagnaro-Green, A., et al. Detection of at-risk pregnancy by means of highly sensitive assays for thyroid autoantibodies. *JAMA* 1990;264:1422–5.

Tunbridge, W. M., et al. The spectrum of thyroid disease in a community: The Whickham survey. *Clin Endocrinol* 1977;7:481–93.

Volpe, R. Autoimmune Thyroiditis, in: Braverman, L. E., and R. D. Utiger, eds., Werner & Ingbar's *The Thyroid: A Fundamental and Clinical Text*. (6th ed. Philadelphia: JB Lippincott, 1981);929.

II. TREATMENT OF HORMONAL IMBALANCES IN FEMALE ALLERGY PATIENTS AT THE HOTZE HEALTH & WELLNESS CENTER

INTRODUCTION

This study was conducted from October 24, 1999, to September 18, 2002, at the Hotze Health & Wellness Center to evaluate the health improvement in female allergy patients who were switched from standard pharmaceutical hormone replacement therapy to bioidentical hormone replacement therapy at their initial visit.

At the Hotze Health & Wellness Center, symptoms of estrogen dominance are treated using oral micronized progesterone in dosages ranging from 6.25 mg to 25 mg twice per day. When estrogen replacement is indicated for symptoms of menopause, Bi-Est is prescribed in dosages ranging from 0.325 mg to 1.25 mg twice per day. All counterfeit hormones are eliminated and are replaced with these bioidentical hormone preparations, produced by a compounding pharmacy.

Patient Population

Total number of female allergy patients treated for
hormonal problems: 269

Number of patients who were premenopausal: 33 (12%)

Number of patients who were postmenopausal: 236
(88%)

Total number of patients responding to questionnaire
about symptoms: 154

Number of premenopausal respondents: 20 (13%)

Number of postmenopausal respondents: 134 (87%)

Average age of premenopausal respondents: 51 years old

Average age of postmenopausal respondents: 57 years old

OVERALL AGE COMPOSITION OF PATIENTS IN THIS STUDY

Premenopausal Patients	Age in Years	Postmenopausal Patients
1	30–39	2
5	40–49	16
12	50–59	67
2	60–69	41
0	70 +	8

Initial Counterfeit Hormone Replacement Therapy in Premenopausal Women

(Some patients used more than one type of HRT)

Counterfeit Estrogen/Progesterone	Number of Patients
Premarin	7
Vivelle	5
Prempro	6
Estratest	1
Estrace	1
Provera	9
Premphase	3
Micronor	3

Average Length of Treatment (Counterfeit HRT)   **4 Years**

INITIAL COUNTERFEIT HORMONE REPLACEMENT THERAPY IN POSTMENOPAUSAL WOMEN

(Some patients used more than one type of HRT)

Counterfeit Estrogen/Progesterone	Number of Patients
Premarin	70
Vivelle	9
Cenestin	7
CombiPatch	2
Prempro	18
Estratest	6
Estrace	10
Climara	4
Esclim	1
FemHRT	4
Provera	9
Activella	1
Ogen	2
Menest	2

Average Length of Treatment (Counterfeit HRT)	9 Years

Results

The chart below summarizes the improvement in symptoms among premenopausal women who were switched from counterfeit hormone preparations to bioidentical hormone replacement therapy. The average duration of treatment with bioidentical hormones in this group was eighteen months.

PERCENTAGE OF IMPROVEMENT AND/OR RESOLUTION OF SYMPTOMS OF PREMENOPAUSAL PATIENTS IN STUDY

Symptom	No. of Patients	Mild Improvement	Significant Improvement	Resolved	Overall Improvement
Low Libido	18	17%	67%	0%	84%
Hot Flashes	13	8%	54%	31%	93%
Fibrocystic Breast Disease	6	17%	17%	33%	67%
Breast Tenderness	11	36%	18%	36%	90%
Night Sweats	10	0%	60%	40%	100%
Endometriosis	1	0%	100%	0%	100%
Ovarian Cysts	1	0%	0%	100%	100%
Premenstrual Headache	5	20%	40%	40%	100%
Irregular Menses	7	14%	29%	43%	86%
Heavy Menses	5	20%	20%	40%	80%
Premenstrual Mood Swings	9	33%	33%	22%	88%
Menstrual Cramping	6	50%	0%	33%	83%
Vaginal Dryness	15	27%	20%	27%	74%
Allergy Symptoms	20	40%	35%	15%	90%

The chart below summarizes the improvement in symptoms among postmenopausal women who were switched from counterfeit hormone preparations to bioidentical hormone replacement therapy. The average duration of treatment with bioidentical hormones in this group was sixteen months.

PERCENTAGE OF IMPROVEMENT AND/OR RESOLUTION OF SYMPTOMS OF POSTMENOPAUSAL PATIENTS IN STUDY

Symptom	No. of Patients	Mild Improvement	Significant Improvement	Resolved	Overall Improvement
Low Libido	112	29%	29%	14%	72%
Hot Flashes	101	12%	30%	47%	89%
Fibrocystic Breast Disease	55	20%	38%	22%	80%
Breast Tenderness	89	20%	24%	49%	93%
Night Sweats	74	8%	32%	57%	97%
Headaches	87	20%	40%	32%	92%
Mood Swings	100	19%	42%	32%	93%
Depression	102	21%	40%	27%	88%
Vaginal Dryness	89	19%	42%	25%	86%
Allergy Symptoms	134	22%	43%	14%	79%

Conclusion

These results demonstrate that female allergy patients, both premenopausal and postmenopausal, who have undergone hormone replacement therapy using bioidentical hormones rather than the counterfeit hormones, experience significant improvement in their overall health and well-being. An overwhelming number of these patients who were treated for their allergies in combination with bioidentical hormones reported a marked improvement in their original symptoms.

REFERENCES

Arafat, E. S., et al. Sedative and hypnotic effects of oral administration of micronized progesterone may be mediated through its metabolites. *Am J Obstet Gynecol* 1988;159:1203–9.

Baulieu, E. E., and M. Schumacher. Neurosteroids, with special reference to the effect of progesterone on myelination in peripheral nerves. *Mult Scler* 1997;3:105–12.

Boosma, D., and J. Paoletti. A review of current research on the effects of progesterone. *Int J Pharm Compounding* 2002;6:245–8.

Boman, K., et al. The influence of progesterone and androgens on the growth of endometrial carcinoma. *Cancer* 1993;71:3565–9.

Cowan, L. D., et al. Breast cancer incidence in women with a history of progesterone deficiency. *Am J Epidemiol* 1981;114:209–17.

Dalton, K. The aetiology of premenstrual syndrome is with the progesterone receptors. *Med Hypotheses* 1990;31:323–7.

Dennerstein, L., et al. Progesterone and the premenstrual syndrome: A double blind crossover trial. *Br Med J* 1985;290:1617–21.

Dennerstein, L., et al. Premenstrual tension—hormone profiles. *J Psychosom Obstet Gynaecol* 1984;3:37–51.

Devroey, P., et al. Progesterone administration in patients with absent ovaries. *Int J Fertil* 1989;34:188–93.

Fitzpatrick, L. A., and A. Good. Micronized progesterone: Clinical indications and comparison with current treatments. *Fertil Steril* 1999;72:389–97.

Formby, B., and T. S. Wiley. Progesterone inhibits growth and induces apoptosis in breast cancer cells: inverse effects on Bcl-2 and p53. *Ann Clin Lab Sci* 1998;28:360–9.

Formby, B., and T. S. Wiley. Bcl-2, surviving and variant CD44v7-v10 are downregulated and p53 is upregulated in breast cancer cells by progesterone: Inhibition of cell growth and induction of apoptosis. *Mol Cell Biochem* 1999;202:53–61.

Graham, J.D., and C. L. Clarke. Physiological action of progesterone in target tissues. *Endocr Rev* 1997;18:502–19.

Gray, L. A. The use of progesterone in nervous tension states. *South Med J* 1941;34:1004.

Greene, R., and K. Dalton. The premenstrual syndrome. *Br Med J* 1953;1:1007–14.

Groswasser, Z., et al. Female TBI patients recover better than males. *Brain Inj* 1998;12:805–8.

Hargrove, J. T., et al. Menopausal hormone replacement therapy with continuous daily oral micronized estradiol and progesterone. *Obstet Gynecol* 1989;73:606–12.

Jiang, C. W., et al. Progesterone induces endothelium-independent relaxation of rabbit coronary artery in vitro. *Eur J Pharmacol* 1992;211:163–7.

Moyer, D. L., et al. Prevention of endometrial hyperplasia by progesterone during long-term estradiol replacement: Influence of bleeding pattern and secretory changes. *Fertil Steril* 1993;59:992–7.

Nilsen, J, and R. D. Brinton. Impact of progestins estrogen-induced neuroprotection: Synergy by progesterone and 19-norprogesterone and antagonism by medroxyprogesterone acetate. *Endocrinology* 2002;143:205–12.

Prior, J. C. Progesterone as a bone-trophic hormone. *Endocr Rev* 1990;11:386–98.

Rylance, P. B., et al. Natural progesterone and antihypertensive action. *Br Med J* 1985;290:13–4.

Sampson, G. A. Premenstrual syndrome: A double-blind controlled trial of progesterone and placebo. *Br J Psychiatry* 1979;135:209–15.

Shi-Zong, B., et al. Progesterone induces apoptosis and upregulation of p53 expression in human ovarian carcinoma cell lines. *Cancer* 1997;79:10.

Shyamala, G. Progesterone action in human breast cancer. 1995. Available at: http://www.ucop.edu/srphome/bcrp/ progressreport/abstracts/patho/lib0448.html. Accessed 1/30/03.

Wright, D. W., et al. Serum progesterone levels correlate with decreased cerebral edema after traumatic brain injury in male rats. *J Neurotrauma* 2001;18:901–9.

Yu, S. et al. Apoptosis induced by progesterone in human ovarian cancer cell line SNU-840. *J Cell Biochem* 2001;82:445–51.

III. Treatment of Low Testosterone Levels in Male Allergy Patients at the Hotze Health & Wellness Center

Introduction

This study was conducted from January 1, 1998, to December 31, 1998, at the Hotze Health & Wellness Center to evaluate the health improvement in male allergy patients diagnosed with hypotestosteronemia (low testosterone levels) who were treated with testosterone supplementation.

At the Hotze Health & Wellness Center, symptoms of low testosterone in men are treated using testosterone cypionate injections.

Patient Population

Total number of male allergy patients diagnosed with hypotestosteronemia: 117

Number of patients responding to questionnaire about symptoms: 87

Number of respondents who were taking testosterone cypionate injections: 61

Average age of respondents: 44 years old

OVERALL AGE COMPOSITION OF PATIENTS IN THIS STUDY

Number of Patients	Age in Years	Average Testosterone Level
5	20–29	15.38 pg/ml
20	30–39	16.43 pg/ml
20	40–49	14.93 pg/ml
11	50–59	12.73 pg/ml
5	60 +	13.74 pg/ml

Results

The following chart summarizes the improvement in symptoms among men taking testosterone cypionate injections as prescribed. The average duration of treatment was 5.4 months. Not all patients had all symptoms; the statistics represent the percentage improvement among patients who initially reported the symptom.

PERCENTAGE OF IMPROVEMENT AND/OR RESOLUTION OF SYMPTOMS OF PATIENTS IN STUDY TAKING TESTOSTERONE CYPIONATE INJECTIONS

Symptom	New Patients 1	Established Patients 2
Fatigue	79% (30/38)	78% (18/23)
Mental Sharpness	81% (29/36)	74% (17/23)
Memory	65% (24/37)	65% (15/23)
Abstract Thinking	69% (25/36)	71% (15/21)
Mathematical Ability	61% (22/36)	55% (12/22)
Goal Setting	66% (23/35)	77% (17/22)
Initiative	86% (31/36)	65% (15/23)
Assertiveness	78% (29/37)	68% (15/22)
Decisiveness	78% (29/37)	70% (16/23)
Sense of Well-Being	84% (32/38)	78% (18/23)
Self-Confidence	76% (29/30)	78% (18/23)
Depressed Moods	71% (25/35)	71% (15/21)
Anxiety	67% (22/33)	65% (13/20)
Irritability	69% (22/32)	65% (13/20)
Insomnia	55% (17/31)	29% (4/14)
Muscle Pain	39% (13/33)	53% (9/17)
Muscle Strength	59% (20/34)	73% (16/22)
Libido	65% (22/34)	77% (17/22)

Total number of new patients: 38 (62%)
Total number of established patients: 23 (38%)

Conclusion

These results demonstrate that testosterone supplementation, when indicated in patients with allergic disorders, provides significant improvement in the patient's overall health, well-being, and energy level. An overwhelming percentage of male patients who were treated for their allergies in combination with testosterone supplementation, when indicated, reported a marked improvement in their original symptoms.

REFERENCES

Bhasin, S., et al. The effects of supraphysiologic doses of testosterone on muscle size and strength in normal men. *N Engl J Med* 1996;335:1–7.

Bremner, W. J., et al. Follicle-stimulating hormone and human spermatogenesis. *J Clin Invest* 1981;68:1044–52.

Finkelstein, J. S., et al. Osteoporosis in men with idiopathic hypogonadotropic hypogonadism. *Ann Intern Med* 1987;106:354–61.

Golden, R. J., et al. Environmental endocrine modulators and human health: An assessment of the biological evidence. *Crit Rev Toxicol* 1998;28:109–227.

Gray, A., et al. Age, disease, and changing sex hormone levels in middle-aged men: Results of the Massachusetts Male Aging Study. *J Clin Endocrinol Metab* 1991;73:1016–25.

Hajjar, R., et al. Outcomes of long-term testosterone treatment in older males. *J Am Geriatr Soc* 1995;43, Supplement.

Horton, R. Benign prostatic hyperplasia: A disorder of androgen metabolism in the male. *J Am Geriatr Soc* 1984;32:380–5.

Irvine, D. S. Declining sperm quality: A review of facts and hypotheses. *Baillieres Clin Obstet Gynaecol* 1997;11:655–71.

Kaiser, F. E., et al. Impotence and aging: Clinical and hormonal factors. *J Am Geriatr Soc* 1988;36:511–9.

Matsumoto, A. M. Effects of chronic testosterone administration in normal men: Safety and efficacy of high dosage testosterone and parallel dose-dependent suppression of luteinizing hormone, follicle-stimulating hormone, and sperm production. *J Clin Endocrinol Metab* 1990;70:282–7.

Matusmoto, A. M. Hormonal therapy of male hypogonadism. *Endocrinol Metab Clin North Am* 1994;23:857–75.

Murray, R. K., et al. *Harper's Biochemistry*. (Appleton & Lang 1990): 516–521.

Nankin, H. R., and J. H. Calkins. Decreased bioavailable testosterone in aging normal and impotent men. *J Clin Endocrinol Metab* 1986;63:1418–20.

Nankin, H. R., et al. Chronic testosterone cypionate therapy in men with secondary impotence. *Fertil Steril* 1986;46:300–7.

Reid, I. R., et al. Testosterone therapy in glucocorticoid-treated men. *Arch Intern Med* 1996;156:1173–7.

Shahidi, N. T. Androgens and erythropoiesis. *N Engl J Med* 1973;289:72–80.

Sonnenschein, C., and A. M. Soto. An updated review of environmental estrogen and androgen mimics and antagonists. *J Steroid Biochem Mol Biol* 1998;65:143–150.

Vermeulen, A. Clinical review 24: Androgens in the aging male. *J Clin Endocrinol Metab* 1991;73:221–4.

Winters, S. J. Current status of testosterone replacement therapy in men. *Arch Fam Med* 1999;8:257–63.

IV. SHORT-TERM TREATMENT OF ALLERGY PATIENTS WITH ADRENAL FATIGUE AT THE HOTZE HEALTH & WELLNESS CENTER

INTRODUCTION

This study was conducted from December 1, 1998, to February 16, 1999, at the Hotze Health & Wellness Center to evaluate the effects of treatment with cortisol in allergy patients who were diagnosed with adrenal fatigue.

At the Hotze Health & Wellness Center, adrenal fatigue is treated using physiologic (sub-replacement) doses of micronized cortisol slow release capsules, produced by a compounding pharmacy. The starting dose is 0.625 mg for children, 1.25 mg for women, and 2.5 mg for men, taken in the morning with breakfast. After two weeks, this dose is doubled.

Patient Population
Total number of patients diagnosed with adrenal fatigue: 149
Number of female patients: 94 (63%)
Number of male patients: 55 (37%)

Total number of patients responding to questionnaire about symptoms: 62
Number of females responding: 40 (65%)
Number of males responding: 22 (35%)

Average age of female respondents: 45 years old

Average age of male respondents: 41 years old

OVERALL AGE COMPOSITION OF PATIENTS

IN THIS STUDY

Number of Patients	Age in Years
1	<10
3	10–19
3	20–29
13	30–39
23	40–49
16	50–59
7	60–69
1	>70

Results

The following chart shows the percentage improvement of symptoms in patients taking cortisol. The average length of treatment was 2.1 months. Not all patients had all symptoms; the statistics represent the percentage improvement among patients who initially reported the symptom.

Percentage of Improvement and/or Resolution of Symptoms of Patients in Study Taking Cortisol

Symptom	New Patients 1	Established Patients 2
Allergy Symptoms	82% (18/22)	44% (15/34)
Asthma	80% (4/5)	50% (6/12)
Recurrent Infections	67% (10/15)	64% (16/25)
Fatigue	91% (20/22)	74% (26/35)
Loss of Appetite	33% (3/9)	24% (5/21)

Total number of new patients: 24 (39%)

Total number of established patients: 38 (61%)

Symptom 2	New Patients 1	Established Patients
Weight Loss	62% (8/13)	17% (5/30)
Abdominal Pain	100% (2/2)	17% (2/12)
Diarrhea	100% (7/7)	33% (3/10)
Low Blood Pressure	100% (3/3)	0% (0/5)
Anxiety	77% (10/13)	48% (11/23)
Depressed Moods	86% (12/14)	62% (16/26)
Irritability	82% (14/17)	59% (16/27)
Restlessness	83% (10/12)	56% (14/25)
Hair Loss	71% (5/7)	31% (4/13)
Joint Pain	91% (10/11)	67% (14/21)
Muscle Pain	80% (8/10)	61% (11/18)
Muscle Strength	69% (9/13)	36% (5/14)
Low Libido	60% (9/15)	37% (10/27)

Total number of new patients: 24 (39%)
Total number of established patients: 38 (61%)

Conclusion

These results demonstrate that natural cortisol supplementation, when indicated in patients with allergies, provides significant improvement in the patient's overall health, well-being, and energy level. An overwhelming percent of patients who were treated for their allergies in combination with natural cortisol supplementation, when indicated, reported a marked improvement in their original symptoms.

About the Author

Steven F. Hotze, M.D., received his medical degree from the University of Texas Medical School in 1976. In the 1980s, he began to explore alternative ways to treat his father's heart disease, searching for real solutions beyond the drugs and surgery that had already failed his father. The safe, effective, nondrug treatments that he discovered enabled his father to live eight more productive years and revolutionized Dr. Hotze's approach to medicine.

In 1989, Dr. Hotze founded the Hotze Health & Wellness Center in Houston, Texas, in order to offer a revolutionary approach to optimal health centered around listening to the patient and providing natural therapies such as bioidentical hormones, allergy immunotherapy, nutritional supplementation, and a balanced, healthy eating program. Over the years, thousands of patients have come to the Health & Wellness Center in order to regain their health and to improve their quality of life.

Dr. Hotze is a fellow member of the American Academy of Otolaryngic Allergy, past president of the Pan American Allergy Society, and founder and president of the American Academy of Biologically Identical Hormone Therapy (AABIHT). Through AABIHT, Dr. Hotze has trained numerous physicians in his proven, effective methods for enabling women in midlife to regain their health, increase their energy, and reclaim their lives.

Dr. Hotze and the other physicians at the Hotze Health & Wellness Center host a radio program, "Health & Wellness Solutions," broadcast in Houston on 700 AM KSEV, Monday through Thursday from 12 noon to 1 pm Central time, and on the web at www.ksevradio.com.

INDEX

Italicized references indicate recipes.

importance of, 5–6
working in pairs, 201–02
and zinc, 225
See also estrogen, testosterone,
  progesterone,etc.
hot flashes, 98, 99, 115, 177
Houston Diagnostic Center, 27
HRT. *See* hormone replacement therapy
Hufnagel, Vicki, 177
hunger, 150, 150 fig 13, 202
hydrogenated oils, 212 fig 21, 215, 215 fig
  22, 237
hyperglycemia, 138
hyperinsulinemia, 203–05, 210
hypertension, 3, 23, 77, 137, 150, 152, 204,
  228, 232
hypochondria, 1, 61, 73, 176
  antidepressant drugs, 10–11
  case study, 9–14
hypoglycemia, 138, 139, 144, 150, 150 fig
  13, 244
hypogonadal, 123
hypotension, 72, 139
hypotestosteronemia. *See* low testosterone
hypothalmus, 68 fig 6, 123
hypothyroidism, 4, 43, 59–83, 98, 131
  and adrenal insufficiency, 135, 138
  and allergies, 69–70
    clinical studies, 309–13
  autoimmune thyroiditis, 69–71, 141, 143
    clinical studies, 309–13
  and basal body temperature, 295
  case studies, 62–64, 82–83, 89–90
  diagnosing, 61
  and heart disease, 76–77
  hormonal imbalance, 2
  and hormone replacement therapy, 111
  questionnaire, 190–92
  symptoms, 71–73
  treatment of, 13
Hypothyroidism: The Unsuspected Illness
  (Barnes), 60
hysterectomy, 34, 89, 92, 96, 121
  and estrogen dominance, 12
  unnecessary, 20, 177
hysteria, 176

I

IgE antibodies, 31 fig 1
immune suppression, 45
immune system, 2, 5, 68, 160, 178, 213,
  221, 244, 247
  and allergies, 30, 31, 32, 35, 37, 41
  and autoimmune thyroiditis, 69
  impairment of, 142, 228
  and yeast overgrowth, 47, 48 fig 2, 49–50
immunotherapy, sublingual. *See* allergies,
  medication for
impotence, 23
indecisiveness, 129
Inderal, 23, 24
infertility, 72, 96, 107, 110, 135, 139
inflammation, 32, 45, 99, 137, 204, 213,
  214, 216, 222
  and cortisol, 137, 142
information from patients as diagnostic
  tool, 36–37
insomnia, 2
insulin, 150, 150 fig 13
  effect of monounsaturated fatty acids, 212
  pairs with glucagon, 202
  ways to keep in normal range, 205–08
insulin-dependent diabetes. *See* diabetes,
  type 1
insulin resistance, 203–05, 210
iodine
  deficiency, 69
  iodized salt, 59
irritability, 124, 127, 129, 208, 246
irritable bowel syndrome, 32
Italian Dressing, Classic, *260*
itching and allergies, 32, 33, 42, 51, 53, 246

J

Jefferies, William McK., 134–35, 140–41
jock itch, 53
John, case study, 38–39
Johns Hopkins University School of Public
  Health, 107, 110
joint pain, 45, 49, 72, 139
Journal of the American Medical Association,
  109, 120–22

recommended for maintaining energy,
250–51
Vegetables and Side Dishes, *270–74*
Vienna General Hospital, 173
Vioxx, 179
viral infections, 33
    and adrenal insufficiency, 135
vitamin and mineral supplementation, 5
vitamin deficiency diseases, 5, 155, 161, 228
vitamins, 144, 155–63, 209, 219–23,
    226–27, 228–29

W

water chestnuts, *277, 291, 293*
water in diet, 152, 153 fig 14, 241, 244
weakness, 159
weight gain, 102, 111, 127, 137, 218
    and estrogen, 96, 112
    and hypothyroidism, 61, 71, 72
    and insulin, 150, 204
    See also obesity
Wellness Revolution, 181–83
WHI. *See* Women's Health Initiative
Whitaker, Julian, 85–86, 89, 156, 219
wild yam cream, 114–15
Willke, Warren, 27
Willoughby, James, 29, 37
women
    and adrenal fatigue, 141–42
    allergies, 85–86
    female traits vs. male, 123
    and hypothyroidism, 70–71, 100
    medical treatment of, 175–78
    postmenopausal, 71, 92, 101, 108–09
    and testosterone, 119–22
Women's Health Initiative, 6, 108–11,
    177–78

X

xenoestrogen, 93, 94, 100, 126
xylitol, 218, 236, 238, 241

Y

yeast, 42, 52 fig 3
Yeast Connection, The, 299
yeast-free eating program, 54–55, 235–45

and restaurants, 242–43
yeast overgrowth, 3, 45–58, 142
    case studies, 47–48, 57–58
    cause of, 57–58
    chronic, 47–48, 57–58
    cycle of illness, 48 fig 2
    questionnaire, 188–89
    symptoms, 45
    treatment of, 14, 51–57
    yeast die-off, 56–57, 239

Z

Ziegler, David, 27
zinc, 159, 161, 220, 225
    Hotze recommended dosage, 225
Zocor, 223
*Zone, The: A Dietary Road Map to Lose
    Weight Permanently* (Sears), 147, 201
zucchini, *273, 284*